The Seeds of Beauty

Defining Your Beauty and Style from the Inside Out

Written by

LAKEYSHA-MARIE GREEN

Drawings by

ALYSE DECAVALLAS

Cover Design by Diala Ali

Author Photo: Michael Sasser

http://www.theseedsofbeauty.com

For Michaela, with love.

THE SEEDS OF Beauty

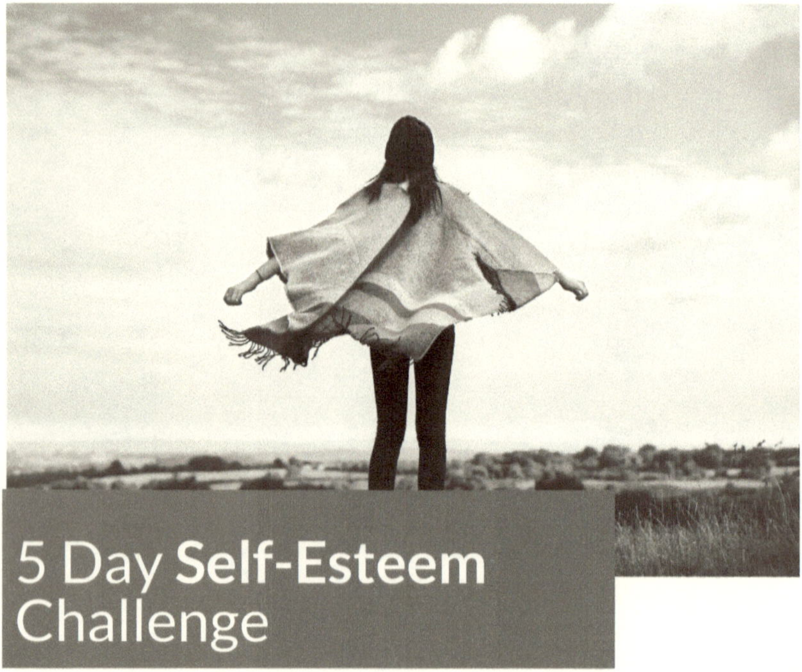

5 Day Self-Esteem Challenge

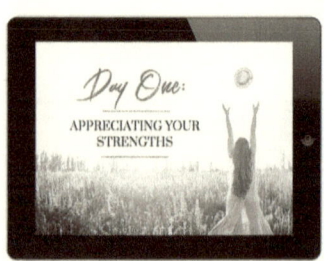

Unlock Your Self-Esteem Daily.

Take the **5-Day Self-Esteem Challenge** today...it's absolutely FREE!

Visit this link to sign up:

www.theseedsofbeauty.com/challenge

CONTENTS

Preface

Worrying, as you know, hardly gets anyone *anywhere*.

So I decided to give my mind a rest for a bit.

I was unemployed at the time and had spent the morning anguishing over when my agent would call with a work offer. "Just breathe," I told myself as I deeply inhaled and then slowly exhaled with a sigh.

To take my mind off things, I decided to accompany my sister and her children while she ran errands. Of course, it's usually when you try to ignore something that it stealthily creeps back into your thoughts. As my sister perused the aisles, my mind slowly drifted back to the stress of my current predicament.

It was then, as I began to feel a rush of despair, that I felt a small, warm pressure against my palm.

Startled, I looked down to discover that my little niece had taken my hand.

At that moment, as I looked into her adoring eyes, the labors of my mind were forgotten. By threading her tiny fingers through mine, she had silently reminded me that there was more to my existence than the anxiety that weighted my spirit. As emotion welled in my eyes, I smiled in awe of the simplicity of the lesson.

No matter who we are, or what our stage in life, we all benefit from reminders of the value and importance of our existence.

As you read each word of Part I: Beauty Within, may it remind you of your worth and the *beauty* that your presence brings into our world.

~Lakeysha-Marie

CHAPTER ONE

The Power of Purpose

"Attain the unattainable."

Tennyson, *Timbuctoo*

Change does not always begin with a well-forged plan from point A to point B. Sometimes change begins with a fleeting thought, a flicker of inspiration, or even a phone call from an old friend to say hello. Then — like a magnet — it draws our thoughts and emotions, inviting excitement with the anticipation of a new life and a new sense of being.

As you begin your journey to further develop yourself, you may find that change is also a little like standing at the beginning of a path with a blindfold on. When you cannot see the path in front of you, it can be difficult to begin the journey. But with a little direction, you will find the courage you need to take that first step forward.

Defining the purpose of this makeover is one of the most important steps of transforming into a more beautiful you. Immersed in the daily expectations of jobs and obligations, we often forget that we too have a voice. And guess what? It *matters*.

By taking the time to identify what you desire to achieve, you mentally create an electric anticipation that will assist you in the pursuit of your transformation goals. In the simplest terms, your aspirations will light the way as you move forward with your evolution. Even though the path can change and veer as you progress, it's easier to take a step forward when you have a vision to guide you.

There was a period when I believed that in order to change my life all I needed was a solid plan. Sounds simple enough, right? After prepping with a few mental side-bends and heart-thumping music to pump myself up, I would sit down to chart out my course of action, only to find a blank white page staring back at me. I was exasperated to find that I had absolutely no idea how to get started.

Why?

A plan simply isn't enough.

Unless you know what you want to get out of your life, or a *vision*, it is very difficult to outline a course of action. No matter how self-assured we are, honestly asking ourselves, "What do I want out of life?" can be the most daunting question of all.

At the age of seven, I was convinced that I wanted to be a baker in a magnificent *pasticeria* when I grew up. Visions of skillfully applying freshly whipped pink icing to a cooled layered yellow cake as the fragrance of warm pastries lingered in the air spilled from my childish mind. Imagine, earning money and eating all the free cake I wanted *all day long* — what more could a sane person want?

Well, seven was a very long time ago. As I grew into an adult and evolved as an individual, I got to know myself better. I found that I wanted more meaningful things like family, great friends, and time to enjoy them. It's no secret that the more you grow and get to know yourself, the more you will discover what you want out of life. So don't feel like you have to have all the answers in the beginning. Just begin by taking time to think about where you would like to be.

Ready to get started?

Close your eyes and visualize yourself peacefully relaxed in your favorite place. Whether it's the feeling of warm sand beneath your feet as you inhale the tranquil saltiness of the sea breeze or nestled snugly in a love-worn chair wrapped in a blanket of bliss, here exists only you and your vision of happiness.

In this place there are no demands with each ring of the cell phone. In this place there is no one present to tell you that you are foolish for hoping for something better. Here, there is not a soul present to remind you of shortcomings. In this moment there is only you and the beauty of everything that is you. As you recline comfortably, focus on what it means for you to be happy with yourself. What does loving and accepting yourself for who you are look like? What does it feel like to you?

Feel the happiness as it courses through you. See the smile on your face as you appreciate yourself. Feel the loving embrace and comfort of accepting yourself as you are and the anticipation of being a better reflection of yourself. Visualize the light within you growing. See it radiating. Watch it wrap itself around you and then around your loved ones. After all, by making the commitment to better ourselves, we in turn better the world and those around us.

It is essential to create a solid foundation upon which to build your dreams. Now is the time to determine the values that are important for your personal success. This is an external exercise as much as it is internal. You will find that surrounding yourself with companions who share your values will create an invaluable positive support system.

When trying to determine what you desire to achieve, you may find it easier to look at your current life and work backwards. Ask yourself, "What do I want to eliminate and *change*?" By eliminating the negatives in your life, you free up more room for the positives to come in.

Beauty Brainstorm:

1. What in your life has led you to make the pivotal decision to begin your transformation?

2. What are the three most meaningful qualities that you wish to develop within yourself?

3. Do you see these present in those with whom you associate and the environments that you function in?

4. If you were to momentarily strip every limitation from your mind and alleviate all traces of doubt, what magnificent things do you see yourself achieving? Imagine if all of your wishes could be granted with the wave of your hand. What is your perfect day? Allow yourself to *dream*.

CHAPTER TWO

Strengthening Your Roots

"Instruction does much, but encouragement everything."

Goethe, *Letter to A. F. Oeser*

It's interesting how you can always sense a subtle shift of mood in the air. It's not always visible, but somewhere within our core we can feel the stirrings of unrest. I could feel it hovering intently as I sat down at the empty table before me.

My palms were damp as I rested my hands on the surface of the table, shadowless from the intensity of the single light that bore down on me. Anxiously peering into the darkness behind the light, my eyes intently searched for the faceless voice that I knew would come.

"How could you be so *stupid*?'

Jumping in my chair, I turned in the direction of the voice.

"It was an honest mistake. I tried my best…" was all I managed to stammer out before the icy voice growled out an abrupt reply.

"That's no excuse — you *know* better! You are a *failure*."

And just like that, as swiftly as it had arrived, the voice was gone and I sat somberly hunched in my chair weighted with the knowledge that I had let myself down *again*.

Why couldn't I get things right? What was wrong with *me*?

Time after time this same scenario would play out, the ruthless inner battle between me and myself. This was long before I realized the power that words held and that when we use them to inflict negativity upon ourselves, we leave behind wounds that cut deeper than the words of another ever could.

Each day many of us awake to the hope of something better. A better life, a better job, a better future. We join the gym and swallow the latest supplements to aid in our endeavor for a healthier life. We go back to school and study tirelessly to earn the degree that will bring the income that we so desperately need to support our families. Countless nights pass by sleeplessly as we push, plot, and plan ourselves to a greater destiny.

Yet when the fruits of our labor and sacrifice arrive as bright and warm as the long-awaited dawn, some of us are greeted by a tinge of sadness in the knowledge that while we have strived and advanced more than we ever thought possible, on the inside we unhappily remain the same.

What was wrong with *me*?

You've probably figured out my problem by now. Despite various accomplishments and personal achievements, the reason I didn't feel good about myself is because I would continually beat myself up over my missteps.

Seems this should be obvious to me, right? Think again. Let's switch roles and then reread the intro. How many times have you come down on yourself unnecessarily only to be later burdened by the guilt and remorse of it all?

As women, we nurture and take care of others whether directly or indirectly. When a loved one has a bad day, we are there to comfort. If our children fail to achieve their set goal, we readily console and reassure them that next time they will do better. But what about us? When we make a mistake, what is the first thing we do?

"I can't believe I did that."

"I'm so stupid."

"How could I have let that happen?"

Immersed in our role as caregivers, we women forget that we have a responsibility to take care of ourselves. We need to be better girlfriends, better wives, and better mothers to ourselves. By fostering a loving and caring relationship internally, we provide the nourishment necessary for our inner beauty to flourish and grow.

It's amazing how deeply we have buried our instinctual resilience over time. As a toddler you learned to walk through a series of falls. Each time you fell, sometimes tearfully but determinedly, you picked yourself up and tried again. It was the fall that taught you to pick yourself up. The end result? You became stronger. Chubby little legs strengthened to provide mobility and tiny feet worked with the brain to ensure you were back on your feet again.

Life, in its unpredictable forms, will present periods where we fall down. It's inevitable. But as adults we tend to forget our resiliency and focus solely on the pain of the fall. Instead of looking for the lesson that will strengthen us and bring us to our feet, we weaken ourselves with self-destructive talk on how we have failed and our disappointment in ourselves. Confidence and assurance are not built by beating ourselves up for making mistakes. These crucial values stem from accepting that things will not always go smoothly and accessing each failure for how it can be better addressed in future.

By doing this, you begin to plant the seeds of inner strength and beauty. Every time you make a mistake is an opportunity to fertilize the soil and strengthen your roots.

In our quest to develop as individuals, one of our first instincts is to list everything that we don't love about ourselves and strategize how to improve.

But what if we instead listed out our *strengths* and reviewed how we can apply them on a grander scale to make our lives better?

Healing and progression typically come quicker when we learn to stop beating ourselves up.

Beauty Brainstorm:

1. When life begins to shift and you stumble and fall as a result of the imbalance, how do you currently handle these obstacles?

2. Reflecting on painful falls of the past, what lessons have you learned that will strengthen your seeds of growth?

3. When you experience the difficult pain of a fall, what are the words that you most need to hear? Write out these words. The next time perfectly articulated plans go awry, gently whisper these words to yourself. True love always begins with you.

4. In your journal, make a list of your personal strengths.

5. How can your strengths be infused into the various facets of your life?

CHAPTER THREE

The Burning Ship

"The virtue lies in the struggle, not the prize."

Richard Monckton Milnes, *The World to the Soul*

On the journey to becoming our better selves, there is always a risk. In essence we are leaving behind the only way we have ever known, however self-destructive it may be. The best analogy I could use here is a burning ship.

Negative thoughts have a way of gaining momentum like a fire stoked by a fiercely moving wind until they quickly surround us with smoke so thick it is hard for us to see through the haze. No matter how much others love us, how many admire us, or how successful our lives may be, we find it harder and harder to breathe.

Trapped on the burning ship that is our inner self, the only way to escape the engulfment is to jump into the water waiting below. The choice to jump can stem from a variety of reasons. It could be a life-changing illness, a divorce from an unhappy marriage, or simply waking up to the fact that we want more for ourselves. Tentatively, we cross the deck and are ready to take the leap. Then, screaming from the abyss of our souls, we take the leap off the ship and land safely into the cool, refreshing waters.

Relieved, we feel the intense sensation of a new start, a new beginning. Happily we laugh as ripples of freedom break through the surface of the water with our every movement. And then the inevitable happens.

We look to the shore and suddenly realize how far away it is. Can we swim that far?

Panic sets in.

We look back at the burning ship and begin to desperately rationalize. Maybe if we splash water on the deck, the flames will retreat and it won't be so bad. Sure, the boat isn't in the best condition, but maybe, just maybe, despite all the holes, it will still make it to shore.

Change can bring a sense of vulnerability to anyone experiencing it. It can be very frightening to step out into new waters. Instinctively, we retreat to what makes us feel safe and secure even if it's a burning ship. Then without realizing it we, like the burning ship, sink back into the same negative patterns of the past. We try to reassure ourselves that it wouldn't have worked out anyway, but in truth we never know because we were too scared to venture beyond our fear.

As you work to better yourself both internally and externally, you may feel the fear that often accompanies change. Like many before you, you will see the distance to the shore and look back to the burning ship. This is a natural reaction that does not indicate weakness.

But instead of returning, you have to make the conscious decision to swim away from the burning ship. With each stroke you will fight the currents of doubt, and each kick will strengthen you and propel you toward your goal. You will tire as everyone inevitably does. But instead of letting yourself sink into the depths of naysayers, float on your back and rest for a bit. Let the waves of hope and the belief in yourself carry you toward shore. And when you are rested and feel strong again, roll over and start to swim again, and don't stop the journey until you reach the shore.

There have been many burning ships in my life from which I have been forced to jump — bad relationships, dead-end jobs, and self-destructive behavior, to name an attractive few.

And because I have the tendency to be stubborn, I have experienced the pain of repeat voyages. How did I learn to stop setting my ships on fire? I began to look for the warning signs. There is always smoke before the flames. When you smell the smoke, which can appear in the form of self-destructive thoughts, insecurities, or pressures to conform to someone else's ideals, stop what you are doing and look to see where the smoke is coming from.

Is this self-induced? Are the people with whom you associate healthy for your well-being? Has someone in the past told you that you weren't good enough, and though buried in the years of your past, the heat of it still burns subconsciously?

If you follow the smoke, you will find the source of your fire. And once you locate it, you possess the ability to squelch it before it turns into a rampant blaze. In doing so you will not only gain insight about yourself, you will also strengthen yourself for the future.

When faced with a hardship in life, it is not uncommon to feel surrounded and entrapped with the emotions of fear, anger, and doubt. However, the next time you feel the four walls around you beginning to inch themselves inward, mentally stand on your tiptoes and peek over the top of the wall to look beyond your current state.

Time keeps moving forward and so will you, even if it's only one small step at a time.

Beauty Brainstorm:

1. Without judgment, pause and take a moment to acknowledge any burning ships that are in your life. Write about each one.

2. Mentally tracing back the smoke, what was it in your life that initiated the blaze?

3. What fears have returned you to the burning ship? Looking back at my voyages, the fear of loneliness as well as unmet expectations contributed to repeat journeys. What are yours?

4. In your journal, describe what you have learned as a result of the hardship. Look for the lesson in everything and remember to keep your focus forward.

CHAPTER FOUR

Bridging the Gap

"To love is human, it is also human to forgive."

Plautus, *Mercator*

In the last chapter, you identified the smoke that aided in the creation of previous fires. The smoke has led you to the initial flames, now what?

What steps do you take to extinguish them?

Start by addressing the source of your fires with forgiveness and acceptance. The past is exactly that—the past. Now is the time, at the beginning of your journey, to have a heart-to-heart with yourself. Address each wisp of smoke with attention and care, as you would with a friend. If you have pent-up feelings or unvoiced thoughts, clear the smoke in the air by writing out those unspoken words or speaking them aloud—even if it's only quietly to yourself. We look so often to others for validation and closure, when in reality true acceptance begins with ourselves.

Let each word fall from your thoughts like droplets of water over the flames until the fire is gently put out. Then mentally open the windows until the smoke begins to clear. With each subtle breeze, feel the negative energy exiting your core and leaving a quiet space for you to reconnect with yourself.

Every time a self-destructive thought enters your head, drawing from the power within you, send a mental love note to yourself to say, "I love you and I accept you as you are." Each time you address a negative thought with love, you weaken its power and in turn positively contribute to your self-esteem.

Fires are destructive in that they have the power to lay waste to even the strongest of structures, leaving behind confusion and feelings of pain. However, each fire also leaves behind a rich soil full of minerals and nutrients that allow us to grow back stronger. In this soil, plant your seeds of beauty and lovingly watch them grow. You will soon find that makeup and beautiful new clothes are no longer tools to cover what you don't like about yourself. They will now be tools to enhance the beauty that is truly your own.

Now is the time for you to make the commitment to evolve into a stronger, more compassionate and beautiful you.

Not ten pounds from now. Not ten years from now. *Right now.*

Since my early years, I have been taught the

importance of forgiveness. The message was as constant as a quiet stream flowing through my life and as essential as breathing. Forgiveness came grudgingly at first, usually following my siblings either taking or breaking my toys. Yet despite the crashing waves of anger that I felt, there was something of a relief in knowing I didn't have to carry around the burden of anger with someone I loved. However, as good as it felt to forgive another, I think the turning point for me came when I learned to forgive myself.

Admittedly, it has been one of the scariest things that I have had to do in my life. It was almost as if it were essential for me to remind myself of missteps in order to make sure they didn't happen again. Could I be trusted not to let myself down in future?

What I failed to realize is that while I had successfully built an emotional nest to seemingly protect myself, the only thing I truly accomplished was clipping my own wings. How can you expect to fly when you are weighted down with chains that hold yourself and your heart to the past?

Have you ever tried to pick up an item when your hands are full? Nine times out of ten you've had to set something down so that your hands were free to take hold of what you wanted to grasp.

Sometimes your heart, like your hands, is filled with thoughts of the past and worries of the future that make it difficult to move forward in the present.

In order to embrace what you truly want in life, it's important to release your grip on the past in order to free up space in your heart.

Here is an affirmation of inner beauty to remind you of the relationship that we must continually build and develop no matter what our stage in life.

Speak the following affirmation of inner beauty aloud until its true meaning resonates within you.

Commitment to Beauty Affirmation

[Your name],

To you, I will never be a fair-weather friend.

When you are afraid,

I will give you the courage to step forward.

If ever you make a mistake,

I will never lose faith in you.

And when you begin to doubt how

beautiful you are, I will remind you.

Today and *every* day

I promise to always stand by you.

You are me. I am you.

I love you.

Beauty Brainstorm:

1. Print out this beauty affirmation from
    http://www.theseedsofbeauty.com and
    carry it with you for the next thirty days.
    Pull it out and let it serve as a reminder of
    how beautiful, resilient, and human you
    are.

2. What wisps of smoke need your loving
    attention? What words have you been
    longing to say? Quietly speak or write these
    weighted words here.

3. Letting go begins with not only accepting
    circumstances, but also accepting your
    emotions. Instead of burying your feelings,
    acknowledge that you are upset,
    acknowledge that you are angry, and
    acknowledge that you are human. By
    releasing these emotions, you free up space
    to heal.

4. Get to the heart of the matter and ask
    yourself, "Why am I holding on to this?"
    Write down your insights in your journal.
    By understanding an underlying issue, you
    can begin to take corrective action.

5. Never underestimate the power of
    forgiveness. Through forgiveness you let go
    of your burden and find strength in the
    wisdom that has taken its place.

CHAPTER FIVE

Finding the Courage to Move Forward

"Push on, keep moving."

Thomas Morton

Healing ourselves and actualizing inner beauty is in many ways no different from learning to walk. It's never an overnight process, but by taking one small step at a time we move closer to our dreams. Often this first step can be as powerful as making a single decision—literally.

There was a period in my life when it was nearly impossible for me to make a decision independently. Don't get me wrong, when it came to addressing problems that others had in their lives I was an expert in providing advice and helpful solutions. I willingly invested the time to listen, console, and give guidance. However, when it came to making decisions in my own life, I was *petrified*.

The extent of this issue did not become evident

until my life had hit rock bottom because I'd failed to take ownership of the decisions that affected my life. I had just ended a turbulent relationship that left me feeling as though the only thing left of my being was a hollow, battle-worn shell. That night as I sat in the dark carpeted hallway and continued to cry the tears that had long ago ceased to fall down my face, I asked myself over and over again,

"How could this happen to me?"

"I'm so smart, how is this possible that I could even end up in a situation as painful as this?"

Have you ever been in a situation where you were left feeling this way? Slowly tracing back the smoke to the start of the blaze, I found pivotal points in time when instead of standing up for myself and being firm in my decisions, I sought to appease. Peering through the smoky haze, I began to see that when we forget about the most important elements that make us who we are, others do as well and treat us accordingly.

It was in that moment I knew I had to change. Anxious but excited, I laid out a plan regarding how I would learn to make independent decisions and gain self-confidence. I would begin by making a decision on my own at least once a week. After assessing my life for any small upcoming changes, I recalled that I needed accessories to finish off a room in my home.

It's so funny the cycles that we get caught in. I remember standing in the middle aisle of the department store fiercely resisting the urge to pull out my cell phone and call someone to help me make a decision about what to buy. I had found a beautiful chocolate-and-bronze tray that I was completely in love with, but I still wrestled with myself mentally.

"What if this is the wrong choice?"

"What if there is something better and I miss it as a result of this decision?"

All of these thoughts raced through my mind until I realized one crucial point. Unless I stopped mentally sabotaging myself with these doubts before I even started, I would never gain the confidence I needed to move forward. So, taking a deep breath, I picked up the tray, walked down the aisle, and approached the counter to make the purchase. Smiling happily and almost tearful, I left the store. For the first time in a very long while I felt a rush of love and pride surge through my heart and even more importantly, I was grateful for the lesson that I had learned.

By taking that little step to progress, I had tapped into the power and beauty within me. I now had something beautiful in my hands to show for it. This, in the simplest of forms, is an example of how by increasing the beauty within ourselves we in turn bring beauty on a physical level into our lives. True style is nothing more than a translation of the beauty contained within. By approaching both our closets and our lives with this mind-set, we mentally prepare for continually putting our best foot forward.

Whether you are just beginning the journey or passing a key milestone, stay motivated by taking one constructive step after another toward achieving your personal goals. Not only will this bring you closer to achievement, it will also serve as a reminder that you are worth everything you wish to obtain.

Beauty Brainstorm:

1. In chapter 1, The Power of Purpose, you made a list of qualities that you desired to develop internally. From this list, select one quality to serve as your starting point. Write it down here.

2. Reflecting on where you currently are in life, what small steps can you take to develop this quality? Draft your plan here.

3. What beauty do you foresee entering your life as a result of the steps that you are taking? How will this benefit you and those whom you love?

4. When your motivation begins to ebb, remember the inspiration for your goal and get excited about the impact you will have!

5. Never give up; you are worth everything that you endeavor to achieve.

CHAPTER SIX

Redefining Your Image

"I am not what I once was."

Horace, *Carmina*

Flipping through an old photo album is one of my favorite rainy-day pastimes. Opening the worn leather cover and brushing my fingers over the thin plastic film that safely holds each memory is like opening a time portal to the past filled with its priceless moments. A slight smile that quickly threatens to become laughter always crosses my face as I glance at the little girl with skinny limbs and thick raven hair. If I knew then what I knew now, how different would my life be?

"Probably boring," I think to myself with a sigh as I turn another photo-filled page. Glancing across the page, my eyes stop at a photo of myself in what I thought to be a very stylish ensemble in my early childhood years. Ever the comedian, I had clothed myself in an oversized plaid trench coat accessorized with scrunched-down athletic socks and white sneakers. I chose to polish the look off with wild hair and a bucket-turned-hat.

Giggling to myself, I wondered what my parents must have thought when they took this photo in our living room so long ago.

Who would have thought this funny little girl would have grown up to be a model and editorial fashion stylist? If nothing else, I suppose it proves the simple fact that not everyone is born with style, *particularly me.*

Much of what I learned and use to help women today was a result of fitting-room trial and error. I had no idea what to wear for my body type, what colors looked good, or even how to apply makeup. As you can imagine, it was a rough and frustrating start, but the more clothing I tried on, the more I began to discover what looked good and what worked best. Slowly but surely, I was transforming into the woman that I wanted be. I discovered that, like many things in life, sometimes you have to try more than once in order to land exactly where you want to be.

Change can be scary at times, but it is also the catalyst that transforms us into everything that we were meant to be. This metamorphosis is such a pivotal moment in our lives and the reason why I enjoy makeovers so much.

The beginning of a makeover transformation is always exciting. I have found that the hustle and bustle of "out with the old and in with the new" ignites inspiration for some of the most fantastic style transformations. However, in the midst of these wardrobe overhauls, I often find that one key element is missing from clothing selections—a woman's goals and dreams.

Our appearance is an expression of who we are and gives the viewer insight into our thoughts, lifestyle, and goals. So it comes as no surprise that a positive personal image is based on incorporating elements of meaning into our look. Fortunately, plugging this piece into the style puzzle is not as tricky as it seems and is something that many of us do without ever realizing it.

When deciding what to wear for a job interview, our first instinct is to read the job description. We scour the professional brief to determine what our prospective role will be and the duties we will be expected to perform. In doing so we ensure that our personal image reflects the goal we wish to achieve, which is getting hired.

Dressing for an interview and dressing for life are no different. By styling ourselves according to our dreams, we are in essence packing our suitcase for the journey and creating continuous motivation.

As you delve into your transformation, it is essential to ask yourself, "How will my appearance reflect who I am and where I want to go in life?" It's important to both mentally and visually align yourself with your dreams from the start, and this begins with reviewing your current wardrobe.

Piece by piece, lay all of your garments and accessories in plain view and again ask yourself, "Do these clothes reflect who I truly am and where I want to go in life?"

As you try on each item, separate your clothing into two piles. Create one pile for "Yes" and the second pile for "No." Return the "Yes" pile to your closet; these items will serve as a foundation for your new wardrobe. Take a look at the "No" pile. Why did you buy these items? Was it on sale? Was it a trend of the moment? Was it a reflection of who you were in the past?

Lovingly bag up the "No" items and drop them off at your local charity shop. Not only are you freeing up room in your own life for positive changes, you are benefiting the life of another woman as well.

After all, when people do good they feel good, and that's a beautiful thing.

Remember that whenever you chart out a course for growth, it's important to set aside time to pause for reflection. It's vital to congratulate yourself on the successes and cherish the wisdom in the moments that didn't quite meet your outlined expectations.

These are the moments within the makeover process when you discover the most about yourself and identify areas that require additional time and attention.

Beauty Brainstorm:

1. Remember the magnificent goals that you wrote about in chapter 1, The Power of Purpose? If your clothing were the words that described to others your most meaningful dream, what items would you choose to wear?

2. Looking at your current wardrobe, do you see elements of your goals and dreams reflected in what you currently wear? When you leave the house, is your outfit purposely put together in a manner that epitomizes who you are as a woman?

3. Complete this exercise by reviewing your wardrobe and creating your own "Yes" and "No" piles. Perform your own act of beauty by donating the "No" pile to someone in need.

4. What have you learned about yourself by completing the above exercise?

5. Describe in your journal your favorite moment so far in your makeover transformation.

CHAPTER SEVEN

Acknowledging Your Value

"The true, strong, and sound mind is the mind that can embrace equally great things and small."

Samuel Johnson, *Boswell's Life of Johnson*

There are words in the English language that are genuinely difficult to pronounce like antidisestablishmentarianism or triskaidekaphobia (a fear of the number thirteen). Yet people go out of their way to learn to pronounce them and even make up silly songs with words that are hard to say, like supercalifragilisticexpialidocious.

On the other hand, the most important things we have to say come with the words that are easiest to pronounce yet we have such a difficult time saying them. Phrases like "I love you" and "I'm sorry" so often seem to get stuck in our throats and never come out of our mouths. The same is true with the simple phrase "thank you." These two words can be so powerful to both the person who speaks them and the person who receives them, and yet we often fail to embrace opportunities to express and receive thanks.

It's not just the grand thanks that are hard to say. Religion has many ways of saying thank you as part of an organized service. Many families incorporate the enumeration of the things they are thankful for as part of their annual Thanksgiving observance. The thank you that is most hard to say is the everyday one, for those little gestures that make our lives more meaningful and enjoyable.

Think about it, when was the last time you said thank you to a clerk at the store who rang your order up without a problem or to a coworker who helped on a difficult project or a loved one for a small kindness that made your day so much better? Did you notice their reactions? Better yet, when was the last time somebody acknowledged an action you took, and how did that make you feel?

You have an immense value as a person that others recognize when they give you a compliment. Accepting their praise and taking it fully into yourself means that you have the ability to acknowledge your own self-worth. You are a good person who deserves to be told how people feel about you. Once you have received that all-important compliment about something you have done or said, accept it with dignity and grace. It is important to say thanks when someone gives you a compliment because it makes both of you feel better.

If you can receive a compliment, it means that you can acknowledge to yourself that you have done something well and are worthy of receiving praise. Saying thank you to people who bestow the gift of a compliment on you says that you value their opinion and tells them that what they say has importance and matters to you.

Like many children, I was taught the importance of showing gratitude for a compliment or kind gesture by saying thank you. Yet, for some reason something strange began to happen. Over time my thank-yous began to evolve into "Oh, it was nothing" or "So-and-so did a better job or "He/She deserves all the credit." How did saying thank you become an afterthought or more importantly, when did it become a phrase so difficult to accept?

When we have low self-worth we may find it difficult to accept praise. We think we are not good enough or are not worthy of this person's acknowledgement of our value. So we try to brush it off with a statement like "Oh, it was nothing special." This confirms to your inner self that you have nothing special to offer and subconsciously says to the other person that he or she is not capable of identifying a special action.

The ability to show gratitude can help you refocus your life from negativity to optimism. Do you see your life as a series of endless tragedies that you somehow deserve? Or have you cultivated the ability to be thankful for those who were there to help you through tough times and thankful that you were able to find the inner reserves to continue on despite what seemed insurmountable at the time? Don't waste time trying to decide whether the glass is half empty or half full; just be thankful that you have a glass and the rest of your life will flow from there.

Try to learn the art of saying thank you again and see what changes it can make in your life and those of the people around you. Start by just making a conscious effort to notice when people do something for you and acknowledge their effort. Then, when people say something nice to you, look them in the eye and simply say thank you.

Don't just say thank you out of habit. Do it in a purposeful way and be genuine in your expression of thanks. As you watch the look of appreciation on the recipient's face, see if you don't just feel a little bit better inside about yourself, too.

Healthy self-esteem stems from acknowledging the value you add to the world.

Beauty Brainstorm:

1. A compliment is a gift. Be appreciative of it by simply saying thank you.

2. Someone else only deserves all the credit if you didn't lift a finger to help. Acknowledge the role you played, however big or small by saying thank you.

3. Share the love. Express your appreciation by giving someone a well-deserved compliment today.

CHAPTER EIGHT

No One Compares to You

"We are such stuff as dreams are made of."

William Shakespeare, *Tempest*

Like skilled artists viewing an amazing piece of artwork, some of us may be captivated and swept away by its glory while others may be swept into a fit of jealousy or envy. Those who fall into the second category are likely suffering from that pesky thing called comparison.

Feelings of insecurity can arise from thinking we'll never be artistic enough to produce a piece of art as wonderful as the one we're viewing.

Unfortunately, our penchant for comparison doesn't stop there.

We compare our hair, weight, outfits, jobs, income, family lives, and even our pets. The comparison factor hits us on all fronts, resulting in emotional turmoil that includes jealousy and anger and can even develop more deeply into hatred or even physical nausea. We'll never win the comparison game, as we will always think someone is younger, thinner, wealthier, more stylish, more happily married, or owns a cuter pet than ours.

Even when we think we've got a heel up on the game by being the thinnest or most stylish or having a happier home life, we still end up losing by putting ourselves above the rest of humanity. Without realizing it, this destroys our connection with our fellows and makes the world a cold, dark, and lonely place. Needless to say, life is not a lot of fun this way.

Even though comparing ourselves to others seems to come naturally, the extent of the habit is not entirely our fault. From the moment we're born we are compared to others and we pick up the habit rather rapidly from there. Parents quickly compare their baby's birth weight, talking skills, and walking age with other children's. Schools reinforce comparisons with gold stars versus the big letter D.

Social protocol hops on the comparison bandwagon with standards dictating that blondes have more fun, Mercedes drivers have more class, and vodka drinkers are wittier than those who drink mere mortal beer. Our culture hails beauty queens and football stars, millionaires and celebrities galore. When we take the comparison route, we believe we'll never be as gorgeous or rich or famous as these folks. Never mind the fact that we never even learned to throw a football or that we may dislike being the center of attention.

With that said, there is a certain level of accountability that we all have for our actions. The responsibility can be placed squarely on our shoulders in two instances. We can take the responsibility for choosing to believe in perceived social standards instead of our own personal truths. We are also accountable when we make unfair comparisons based on those other nasty things called "shoulds."

We might think we should be the next Picasso, Vivaldi, or Einstein even though we neither practiced nor developed artistic, musical, or mathematical skills. Why we think we should be the best at everything may remain a mystery in its origins, but its outcome is blatantly clear: "shoulds" can quickly fuel us with jealousy and the feeling of being less-than.

It's no surprise that comparison can spark within us negative emotions, but that's nothing compared to what it does to our self-esteem. Comparison annihilates it. It's tough to feel good about ourselves, after all, when we believe that whatever we think, whatever we do, and however we look will never measure up to someone else.

Instead of celebrating the strengths and assets we do have, we instead focus on those we may never attain. We become stifled by self-loathing and shame. As time progresses we become further ashamed of who we are because the way we actually see ourselves is so far removed from what we think or wish we could be.

We can only restore our self-esteem and feel good about ourselves if we accept ourselves as we are. Each person is wholly unique and each comes with his or her own unique strengths and weaknesses. Accepting both the strengths and weaknesses gives us the humility we ultimately need to forge a true bond with our fellows as well as the boost we need to feel good about ourselves. In doing so, we create a healthy and positive self-esteem.

Once we view ourselves honestly, without the distortion of comparison, we can begin to enjoy and actually love ourselves. Jealousy, rage, shame, hatred, and even nausea can dissipate nearly instantly — although accepting ourselves as we are may take a bit of practice. Therefore, be prepared to provide yourself with both patience and time to fully heal.

The trick is to stay on top of it, to recognize when the comparison factor begins to set in so we can stop it in its tracks. Rather than lamenting that we'll never be as artistic as Picasso or as musically inclined as Vivaldi, we can try focusing on our skill at turning any recipe into a great work of art, our ability to play a mean ukulele, or whatever other talents and strengths we do have.

Only when we stop trying to measure up to someone else or the warped set of ideals set by external factors can we truly become and enjoy the beautifully unique individuals we were meant to be.

Always remember that when you begin comparing yourself to others, you immediately put yourself at a disadvantage. Everyone has unique talents, experiences, and stories that make them who they are.

It's what makes you truly beautiful.

And *nothing* compares to that.

Beauty Brainstorm:

1. When you begin to compare yourself to someone else, silently pause and redirect your thoughts.

2. Write in your journal the top ten things that you love about yourself.

3. Self-love is not conditional. Love yourself for your strengths and your weaknesses. It's the powerful union of the two that make you who you are.

CHAPTER NINE

Facing Your Fears

"The lofty oak from a small acorn grows."

Lewis Duncombe, translation of *De Minimis Maxima*

Growing up, I was never a fan of scary movies. Even as an adult, I have no shame in telling you that the eerie crescendo of the violins and rapidly increasing thump of the drums were my cues to shut my eyes and subtly extend my fingers to cover my ears. In other words, keeping my eyes open during a scary movie is a lot like trying not to blink when there's dust in your eye—not going to happen.

Of course, this would all quickly change.

Whether on screen or off screen, fear has a funny way of inhibiting our understanding when we allow it to take control. In this instance I continually missed pivotal parts of the narrative that pulled the film together. Annoyed with my questions of "What happened?" each time I reopened my eyes, my sister determined enough was enough.

During the film as if perfectly timed, she ripped my hand from my eyes precisely when another hideous being appeared. With little choice in the matter, I was forced to face my fear in all of its horrifying Hollywood glamour. A few seconds passed and after facing the would-be gremlin, I found I still had ten fingers and ten toes. Needless to say I quickly realized that I had nothing to be afraid of. Laughing to myself, I began to ponder this lesson on a bigger scale.

How many times in life do we mentally cover our ears at the sound of a new idea because it makes us uncomfortable? Or how often have we closed our eyes out of fear of challenges that unexpectedly appeared in front of us? When we succumb to the things that make us afraid, we limit our opportunity for growth and inhibit a deeper understanding of the plot unfolding before us.

However, when we open our eyes to face our fear, we are in a position to not run from it but walk *through* it.

One of the scariest things I have ever had to do was learn to let my guard down and open up to those around me.

Growing up I was a very shy and self-conscious child. As you can imagine, if something went wrong it did not take much for me to feel uncomfortable or embarrassed. It was a sensitivity that often left me feeling as though I continually came up short, when in reality nothing ever goes according to plan and part of growing is making mistakes. As I grew older I made the decision to separate myself from this sensitivity by disregarding these emotions. After all, if you don't acknowledge it you don't feel things, right?

Wrong.

But more on that later.

I became quite good at masking my feelings of pain and embarrassment. Anytime a situation occurred that I was uncomfortable with or made me feel as though I were on the spot, I would simply take my emotions and mentally tuck them away behind a wall. It became my little barrier of protection and with each stone that was placed the wall became stronger. My confidence grew and I also felt resolute in knowing that nobody would be allowed to hurt me or get me down. This was something that I could control. The threat of pain was now a thing of the past. The whole sticks-and-stones concept was moving along swimmingly.

But as you know, few things come without consequences, and my stony cobbled wall was no exception.

You see, when you build a wall to prevent things from getting in, this also prevents things in the inside from *going out*. I struggled immensely with the ability to honestly express my intimate thoughts and emotions. Anytime I attempted to do so I felt so open and exposed. It was as if I was laying myself at the feet of wolves and I was the delectable rabbit. The vulnerability left me feeling unprotected and scared me immensely.

However, as scary as it seemed, I knew that I would have to face my fears if I were ever to have deeper, more meaningful relationships with anyone. Instead of burying my feelings, I needed to find a way to acknowledge them and then let the emotions go in a way that was constructive to my self-esteem.

I began slowly by verbalizing the emotions I felt as they began to surface. The start was anything but graceful. I would start speaking then stop, fumble over my words and lament over if I were actually getting my point across. Yet the shell of the acorn had begun to crack and as time passed my roots took to the earth and I became better at communicating my feelings, which in turn made me stronger.

The biggest surprise for me was the more I shared myself with others, they in turn shared themselves with me. It was almost as if being myself let others know that it was okay to do the same.

As the blossom grew into a flower, it wasn't always a bed of roses. More than once someone came with an axe and struck it against the trunk of my tree. And while it wounded the surface and the blade sometimes went a little deep, it wasn't enough to break me because I was not the same person that I used to be. Through facing my fear, I had become stronger.

Now, nowhere does it say you won't have butterflies in your stomach or moist palms, so it's safe to assume that's okay. After all, there is nothing wrong with being afraid. The problem comes from letting the fear stop you from becoming everything that you were *meant* to be.

So the next time you find yourself feeling afraid, acknowledge it. Then take a deep breath, peel your fingers from your eyes, and move forward.

Who knew you could be so brave?

Beauty Brainstorm:

1. Draw the outline of a tree in your journal and write your name at the base of the trunk.

2. On each branch write a different answer to the following question: "What would I achieve if I weren't afraid?"

3. This tree represents only a sliver of everything that you have the potential to achieve. By moving beyond the limitation of fear and doubt, you awaken the powerful potential that you have within.

CHAPTER TEN

The Problem with Perfection

"It takes two to speak the truth — one to speak, and another to hear."

Henry David Thoreau

"Would you rather be right or would you rather be happy?" It's a question that has swirled in the minds of all people at some point in time. It is a question frequently broached by marriage or relationship counselors as well as parents, friends, and coworkers. The driving desire and need to be correct at all times leaves deep imprints in each person's relationships and has reached nearly all levels of our daily interactions.

Often, issues of right and wrong are closely tied with a personal sense of identity. They represent the key blocks in the building of the ego. Think about it. You feel satisfied when everyone acknowledges that you're right. When you are wrong, it is not uncommon to feel embarrassed or even humiliated.

However, at times we can have such a desire to get ahead in the race that we do not stop to think about the possible downfalls that can occur from insisting on being right. In the minds of many individuals, one *has* to be right because the alternative is to be wrong, and people who are wrong are not going to advance.

These ideas of being right versus being wrong can be seen as early as the school classroom. Teachers praise students for coming up with the right answer, which often quickly leads to other awards and prizes. In school, I remember having the belief that students who are able to come up with the correct answers frequently will go on to achieve higher grades, attend good colleges, and obtain good jobs. They will get ahead in life.

This sense of achievement carries through to adulthood, where people seek to get ahead in their jobs and other areas of their lives through being right, having already firmly absorbed the cultural belief that being right brings reward and satisfaction.

However when we insist on only being right we often find ourselves facing a number of social difficulties. People who continually fight every point find themselves annoying and pushing away many people in their lives such as family members, friends, and spouses. Not to mention people in general are not fond of being corrected or argued with on a regular basis. If one person in the relationship is also firmly entrenched in the need to be right always, the battles between the two individuals can get very deep.

Insisting on being right is also a source of unnecessary stress. When we focus such a large part of our energy and identity on being right, the threat of being wrong can be debilitating.

If our sense of value and worth is centered on our ability to be right all the time, when we are wrong we are left with nothing.

It's a lonely feeling that many of us go to extremes to avoid. When arguments arise, we feel all the typical symptoms of stress, such as sweaty palms and a quickening heart rate. Somehow it becomes easier to ignore the repercussions of our actions than to have to look at ourselves in the mirror and accept that we were incorrect.

But what if we took the time to step back and be human? What if we instead saw being wrong for what it truly is—an opportunity to learn and grow? After all, it's difficult to understand the lesson without first listening to the teacher.

Allowing ourselves to be open to the idea of being wrong lifts a large stress off of our hearts. We will no longer have our personal identity tied to this need to be correct. This will allow us to build relationships on a much deeper level and learn to better understand the perspective of another. By ridding ourselves of embarrassment associated with being wrong, we actually become *stronger* because we have less to fear.

Letting go and allowing ourselves to be wrong enables us to learn and develop on an entirely different level. It allows us to adapt our understanding of ourselves and the world and move forward more enlightened beings. Without the need always to be right, you make room to build admirable traits such as empathy, courage, and imagination.

When we are able to admit when we are wrong and forgive others who do the same, our relationships are enriched through the mutual act of speaking and listening.

Listening to the opinions of others is also a good way to facilitate fruitful discussion. When you show interest and respect in another's opinions, it is natural for the other to reciprocate, which leads to an open and engaging conversation that can generate interesting ideas.

Mutual respect and appreciation is essential for developing valuable interpersonal relationships. Listening can also enable people to consider topics in ways they may not have previously considered, allowing them to grow in their knowledge.

In the heat of an argument, it's hard to fight the temptation to secure the title of being right. Yet, sometimes earning that title can do us more harm than good. Though we will not always see eye to eye in the ring, it's important to both acknowledge and respect each other's stance.

Remember, the need to be right isn't always right. Sometimes, it's more important for someone to hear that you simply *understand*.

One of the few things stronger than being right is the power to gracefully admit when you are wrong.

Beauty Brainstorm:

1. Being right all the time is a heavy burden to carry. Free yourself of the sagging weight by admitting, "I don't know" or "I was wrong."

2. When left unchecked, fear and ego can cloud our judgment. Ask yourself, "Why do I feel the need to be right?"

3. Lay the groundwork for compassion by reminding yourself that while you don't necessarily agree with the other person's conclusions, it's important to take the time to listen.

CHAPTER ELEVEN

It's Your Time

"Time is the life of the soul."

Henry Wadsworth Longfellow, *Hyperion*

As the dawn slowly broke, washing the gray-and-brown rooftops of the sleeping city in a soft amber light, I stirred suddenly and then quickly arose from bed in anticipation of the day ahead. Today I had been booked to style an edgy yet soulful emerging artist and his band for a music video shoot to debut their latest track. Like many projects, this was not the standard run-of-the-mill call your agent and book. In fact, at the time I had no agent and the booking had been a result of a chance encounter over a drink with friends. Still, it was paying work and based on my lean account balance, I could really use the boost.

With the final touches of my DVF berry-hued lipstick applied, I confidently walked out the door and headed to the studio. Upon arrival to the set, the air was electric with the hum of conversation and movement. Black cords wound along the floor and intertwined like dropped spools of ebony thread, and I silently thanked the little voice of reason for suggesting that I not wear heels today.

After checking in with the production team, I was led to a small area where my rails and clothing had been deposited. Next to me were the makeup artists who skillfully worked on the backup singers who both greeted me warmly with smiles. No egotistical divas. Relief flooded me and internally I beamed. Today was going to be a good day.

Despite arriving to the set early, there was much to be done and it was not long before the shouts of the producer directing the team could be heard. This was a new client for my portfolio and the last thing I wanted to do was fall behind. Fashion styling is a competitive business, and a successful shoot could mean repeat business. I recognized the advancing shuffling of footsteps signaling the arrival of the band, and I felt a small panic starting to build in my chest. Just breathe, I told myself. I silently willed the steamer to begin puffing mists of heat to smooth the travel-creased garments that hung impatiently on the hangers. I decided to distract myself by prepping the outfits for the singers who were having their final touches of powder applied. As if on cue I heard a stern voice ring out, "We need to start dressing the backup singers!"

Belting out a reply, I hastily turned and was stopped dead in my tracks by the contact of my forehead with the blunt end of the clothing rack.

Reeling from the blow, I instinctually looked around to see if anyone had noticed.

Clearly, my vanity had not suffered.

Peering out into the swirl of the crew's choreographed chaos, it was evident that in the wave of barking orders, my accident had gone unnoticed. Touching my throbbing forehead, I closed my eyes in silent relief and in the quiet I heard a small voice whisper, "Slow down."

After filling my lungs with a deep breath, I slowly exhaled to clear my mind of the anxiety that clouded it. As the corners of my lips turned up into a sympathetic smile, it occurred to me that when we lose ourselves in the manic shuffle of time, we weaken the strength of our mental focus and concentration. This in turn inhibits our ability to be the best we can be at the task at hand. Whether it's getting through a demanding day, or in my case styling a photo shoot, when stress and worry is allowed to dominate our lives we automatically place ourselves at a disadvantage. Often, as was the case in my story, we can even cause mental or physical injury to ourselves in the process.

Therefore, if ever you find yourself in a moment of panic or frustration over how you will make it through one of life's curveball scenarios, it is imperative that you take a moment to slow down and refocus. Remember, each day is filled with the same amount of time as the last and what counts is not how quickly it goes by or seemingly slips through our fingers but how we direct each moment.

Turning around, I began styling the waiting performers and as time steadily wound its way through the day, I quickly but clearly pulled each outfit together. Pretty sequined dresses were fitted on the singers, suspender straps were adjusted to suit varying heights of the band, and with each snap of a button I felt myself growing more assured.

By the end of the shoot I was exhausted, but as we all stood together to pose for a production team photo it was impossible not to smile. While the start of the day was tumultuous, it ended in a lesson of how not to get lost in the shuffle of time and the importance of realigning yourself in the midst of chaos.

In a swiftly moving world centered on the tick-tock of the clock, time seems more of an elusive phantom than an ever-present friend.

While you cannot slow the minute hand as it methodically moves throughout the day, you do possess the pivotal power to make every moment count.

Picture yourself using time to not only hear but to listen.

Imagine taking the time to not only accept but to thoughtfully appreciate.

And above all, remember what it feels like to take time for you.

Beauty Brainstorm:

1. Review this week's calendar and schedule a date with *yourself*. Whether it's watching a movie or buying something special, a little "me time" is essential for well-being.

2. Begin every day this week with purpose. Each morning, set one important task that will bring you fulfillment to accomplish.

3. Every night before going to bed, take a moment to reflect on your day. In your journal, describe your favorite part of each day as well as any lessons or "ah-ha" moments that you observed.

CHAPTER TWELVE

The Defining Moment

"Our growing thought makes growing revelation."

George Eliot, *Spanish Gypsy*

It is said that honesty is the best policy, so when it comes to my hair I will be the first person to admit to you that I am a commitmentphobe. *Seriously.* Whether I wear it long, cut it short, dye it black, or highlight it caramel brown, it seems that no hairstyle is ever enough to satiate me for more than a few months. But change is a good thing, right?

As I pondered this thought, my mind drifted to a friend who frequently wore her jet-black hair in long micro braids that curled slightly where they ended above her waist. I remember when I first saw them I was immediately transported back to my childhood, when my mother would spend hours braiding my hair into intricate styles that would last for weeks at a time with proper upkeep. It was an amicable compromise between taming my abundantly thick hair into submission and her sanity as a mother.

Excited, I approached my new companion with questions on where she had her hair done and how often she cared for it. As you can imagine, it wasn't long before I too had a head full of bouncy braids in a golden-brown hue. I had gone to the beauty supply shop and purchased beautiful brown extensions that the hairstylist artfully blended into the braids with my natural hair for a stunning finish. When my friend saw my new hair she was elated, and after pausing to admire she leaned close and whispered to me, "Are those extensions?"

Laughing, I replied, "Yes."

She then asked, "Don't you feel fake?"

Turning to her in surprise, I responded, "No, why?"

She went on to explain that whenever someone asked her if she wore extensions, she felt insecure and fake because it wasn't her natural hair. I stared at the beautiful woman before me in disbelief. In listening to her, I began to see that there was a disconnection within her between her outer appearance and her inner beauty.

Instead of channeling her beauty from the inside out, she was channeling from the outside in. The opinions of others seemed to silently guide her self-esteem and as a result, instead of the braids being an extension of her natural beauty, they had become an area of sensitivity that adversely affected her self-image.

Working behind the scenes of photo shoots where I change a model's look at the drop of a hat with everything from wigs to "chicken cutlets," I was slightly baffled by her reply. I went on to explain to her that whether we change our hair from short to long, gray to blonde, the authenticity of our character lies within our heart and spirit. These are the elements that encompass our beauty and make us who we are.

Inner beauty is a reflection of love and like its counterpart it begins at the heart of things, *from within*. One of the most valuable and sometimes painful lessons that we learn in relationships is that it is difficult to fully love someone without first knowing what it means to love yourself. Sure, you can make it a good distance at the beginning, but eventually the empty space that you wish to fill, will begin to swallow up and destroy all that you have sought to create.

In order to share love with another, it must first exist within you, otherwise you have nothing to contribute and enrich your partner. Ultimately anything that you seek to build without a foundation will inevitably collapse.

Developing inner beauty is no different in this regard. When we rely solely on external sources such as compliments and attention to make us feel beautiful and worthy of existence, we are only as good as the last pleasantry spoken to us. Thus the distance between an admiring glance and words of adoration can lead us to feel insecure and doubt who we are at the center of our being.

Making the shift from channeling your beauty from the inside out is a little like changing a blown light bulb. In order to regain your source of light, you must first replace the bad bulb with a good one.

Whenever a negative self-image enters your mind, calmly acknowledge it and say, "Okay, it's time to change the light bulb."

As you climb the ladder to the fixture, remember to take a slow, deep breath. Mentally unscrew the darkened bulb with the energy of a positive thought.

Then flip the switch and let your inner light shine.

What defines us isn't contained in a box of Clairol, the silky strands of extensions, or apparel from the latest designer collection. These are all external components whose purpose is to enhance the true beauty of a woman, not define it.

When shopping for new ways to make over your look, always remember the purpose behind the product. Every product you purchase, whether it's a beauty cream, new dress, or pair of shoes, should only have one end goal, and that is to enhance the natural beauty that is already your own.

Look for silhouettes that flatter your body line, cosmetics that enhance the natural color of your eyes, and flattering hair colors that radiate against your complexion. In doing so you are channeling from the inside out and creating a new look that's all your own.

And there's *nothing* fake about that.

Beauty Brainstorm:

1. In your journal, write down every wonderful blessing present in your life. From a home to a family, remind yourself of the blessings you have to keep negativity at bay.

2. For the duration of this week, practice using only positive words when describing yourself to others.

3. Be aware of your thinking and change the light bulb when needed to improve your well-being and let your inner beauty radiate.

CHAPTER THIRTEEN

A Perfect Fit

"We know the truth, not only by the reason, but also by the heart."

Blaise Pascal, *Thoughts*

"Tonight I am going to meet him," I thought to myself as I slowly turned from the window. The growing pile of clothing next to my bed representing my indecisiveness wasn't altogether encouraging, but I was still in good spirits.

Smiling, I stole a sip from my glass of wine to calm the butterflies that danced in my stomach. This was my first date in a long time and I really wanted to make the right impression. Walking over to the wardrobe, I opened the wooden doors as I wondered what I should wear.

Slowly, I ran my hand over the racks, feeling the textures of the dresses beneath my fingers. What to wear? Glancing at the clock, I quickly pulled out three dresses and laid them across my bed to try on.

The first dress was a style I'd purchased with a friend. The sleek cut of the metallic fabric was contoured and modern—a little daring to some but right on trend. As the steel-hued dress slipped over my head, I smiled and turned to the mirror in anticipation. To the naked eye, it was perfect.

However, as I stepped closer, I noticed it fit beautifully at the waist but the shimmering fabric just didn't lay flush against my heart. Taking a step back, I took in the extraordinary color as I stood under the light, but like a forced smile, its radiance didn't quite reach my eyes.

Why did I get this dress again? Ah yes, this dress was my way of seamlessly blending into the social circle. Looking down, I noticed a few loose sequins that left a visible scar along the surface of my skin during wear. Mentally wincing, I recalled the discomfort that often accompanies not being myself.

The next dress I tried on was a gift from my parents. It was conservative in style but sophisticated and very beautiful. The soft fibers of the materials spun together family values that were accented with pearls of firm direction. Maybe it was the little bit of weight I'd put on as I grew over the years, but it felt very constricting. While I felt safe and secure with each sweep of the skirt, I heard the threatening tear of the seams as I attempted to zip the back of the dress. Sighing to myself, I realized that it was time to let this one go. As much as I loved this dress, it was time for me to grow into something that was more of my own.

The third dress was an equally gorgeous shade of icy blue, but the weight of the fabric made it heavy and cumbersome. This dress had seen a lot of wear in my last relationship. The crease was still visible from where it had been pressed tirelessly to be worn in perfection. Turning in the dress, I saw the various areas where I had so desperately tried to mend it. So many times I had attempted to wash out the dirt of a relationship stained with distrust. Looking at my reflection, I saw the broken stitches between us that I had tried so hard to keep together. As the emotion rose to the surface, I wondered why I had even kept this dress after all the pain it caused me.

In all honesty, I had been afraid. Every time I went to throw it out, I thought, "I can tailor the fit. Maybe use the fabric for another dress and repurpose it." When in reality what I needed to do was let it go. Taking a deep breath to steady my shaking hands, I bravely ripped the dress in two. Each tear of the material seemed to free me from the threads that had invisibly kept me tied down. Even though it felt good, I noticed that I was a little sad afterward and I *still* had nothing to wear.

Feeling the anxiety building, I was about to burst into tears when something caught my eye. In the back of the closet was a box tucked amongst the shadows of old things. Blowing the dust from the lid, I carried the box to my bed and opened it. As soon as I pulled out the dress I recognized it immediately. It was a deep red that spilled across my hands into a pool of burgundy material as it caught the light. Despite its age, the dress appeared nearly brand new as it was rarely worn over the years.

Holding it up for examination, I saw the delicate stitching of dreams long ago carried in my heart. And though barely visible to others, I saw the patches that had been applied to the hem from falls I'd taken while walking on the unpredictable road of life. Though old, it was beautiful and I wondered to myself why I never wore this dress — a dress that was so close to me and I knew so well.

Then I remembered.

I had been so busy trying on new dresses to stay on trend and fit in that I had discarded this dress, *my dress*, in the process.

After pulling the dress over my head and twirling to face the mirror, I paused to look at my reflection in the long mirror.

"Finally," I said as I sighed happily.

A perfect fit.

Strength and beauty is facilitated by living and speaking your inner truths, not those of others.

If ever you find yourself sliding into the trap of telling someone what they want to hear, take a step back and ask yourself, "Are the words I am about to speak of truth?"

By speaking in honesty and being true to your values, you give others the permission and courage to do the same.

Beauty Brainstorm:

1. Ask yourself again, "What are the values that are most important to me?"

2. In your journal, list any areas where you tend to struggle with honesty. What hinders honesty in these areas? Is it fear? A method of distraction?

3. What constructive steps can you take to address the root of the problem to ensure you align with your values identified in question one?

CHAPTER FOURTEEN

Discover and Define Your Style

"Love does not dominate, it cultivates. And that is more."

Goethe

Um…exactly who are you again? Whether it's jeans and a tank or a couture cocktail dress, stunning style begins with you. After all, style is nothing more than an expression of who you are as a person. Think of it as a spotlight that highlights and enhances your identity as you take to the stage of day-to-day living. For this reason it's important that your style truly reflects your individuality. Otherwise, someone else might be stealing the show.

Now before you roll up your sleeves and begin pondering the age old question of "Who am I?" let's put this into perspective.

At some point in your life, you probably closed your eyes and wistfully envisioned the person that you wanted to be. Perhaps it was an athlete, a businesswoman, a teacher, or a mom. Whatever it was, there was something special about this image that connected to you.

Maybe it was the surge of adrenaline from winning a championship that inspired you or the authoritative role of leading a board meeting to shape the direction of a company. It may be that you've always had a knack for helping others to understand complexities or perhaps nurturing has always been second nature to you.

Similarly, your personal image is in many ways as much an emotional connection as it is a visual one. How you feel about yourself emotionally and how you wish others to perceive you often affects your everyday appearance. So it comes as no surprise that at the beginning of your makeover journey, the most important question you can ask yourself is "How do I envision myself?"

Why?

How you envision yourself is the baseline for every decision you make in your life, *including* what to wear. Nine times out of ten if you envisioned being an athlete, you weren't running down the track in a tutu, and more likely than not your tee-and-yoga-pant combo didn't make it into the board room. That's why it is essential to understand what defines you as a person in order to define your style.

So, let's get started.

Step 1:

Start by taking a moment to envision yourself as you are at present. This isn't the new you after the promotion, after losing ten pounds or, my personal favorite, post lotto winnings. This is you in your day-to-day life — going grocery shopping, at work, walking the dog, running a business. Pay attention to the clothes you have on and the colors you wear. How's your hair looking today? Any makeup on?

As these images begin to build in your mind, write them down. At the end you should have a brief description of how you see yourself right now.

Step 2:

Now that you've got your brain warmed up, how do you envision your life as a result of your makeover? This is *your* transformation, so have fun with it. What shoes are you wearing? What job do you see yourself acquiring? Did you cut your hair? Are you wearing a new color? Getting married?

Step 3:

Once you have completed the description of step 2, place it next to the description from step 1. Take note of the differences and similarities between the two descriptions. Jot down what you discover. By pinpointing the differences, as well as consistencies, you will begin to see the tiny elements that we'll later use to define your style.

How?

Glad you asked. Most women are a combination of styles; however, there are key dominate traits in every woman that make her look unmistakably distinct. These traits have been grouped into six categories:

Classic. Classic women have timeless looks that never go out of style. They prefer to dress in silhouettes that create a clean, smooth line. Although they may not follow every trend, they pick up fashions of the moment in the details of their accessories. Classic color selections include blue, khaki, black, and white.

Dramatic. Dramatic women prefer vivid colors and patterns that catch the eye. They love to dress in cuts and silhouettes that flatter the figure for a striking appearance. Creativity is their anthem and is reflected in their makeup and hair styles.

Elegant. Elegant women enjoy creating looks that are polished and classic. Quality fabrics and clean lines play a key role in their style choices. Subtle ruffles and feminine details can be found in their wardrobe, but nothing too extravagant or over the top.

Natural. For the natural woman, comfort reigns supreme when selecting clothing. Fabrics that move freely with the body in carefree colors and earthy prints give a bohemian air to her look. Simple hair and makeup characterize her, highlighting her natural beauty.

Romantic. Sugar, spice, and everything nice.

Romantic women create looks that are soft and feminine. Satins, lace, and flirty trims are sprinkled throughout their wardrobe. Soft makeup and pastel colors contribute to their ambiance of romance and love.

Sporty. Smart trainers, cropped trousers, and vintage tees. Whether dressed up or down, sporty women prove that it's possible to dress comfortably and still look great. Simple hairstyles, whether cropped or pulled back, complement their look and makeup is usually minimal.

Take both descriptions from steps 1 and 2 and compare them to the style profiles above. What similarities do you see between what you envisioned and the descriptions provided?

To which style do you connect most closely?

Once you determine the style that best aligns with who you are as a person, you can then begin shopping for clothing and accessories that match it.

After all, this is who you are.

This is your life.

Go for it.

Beauty Brainstorm:

1. Using this guide, which style do you most identify with the most?

2. Can you see parts of yourself in any of the other personal style descriptions? Which ones?

3. Does your current wardrobe reflect your style personality?

PART II:

Beauty Reflected

Beauty Reflected Introduction

It's no surprise that your physical appearance is a direct extension of the beauty residing within you. When you are imbalanced with the weight of low self-esteem and feelings of inadequacy the burden is visible in your body language and appearance.

That's why before the swipe of the credit card, or snip of the shears, every makeover transformation begins with a reconnection to who you are at your core. In Part I, Beauty Within, you joined me on an intimate journey that unveiled the essentials for creating self-love and confidence. Now, it's time to take the beauty that defines you on the *inside* and incorporate it into your personal style.

Through my own fashion *faux pas* I've learned that dressing well requires a clear understanding of the fashion and style fundamentals. Fashion trends continually flow in and out, switching like the tides. However there are beautiful classics such as the little black dress that defy the waves of time.

In Part II, Beauty Reflected, you will find core fashion basics to either begin your fashion makeover or simply update your current style. As you read be conscious of how each skirt, dress and shoe fit into the frame of how you picture yourself to be. Your goal is to take the patterns, textures and embellishments that reflect your personality and incorporate them into silhouettes and colors that best suit your body shape and complexion.

If you find that you gravitate towards a specific color, ask yourself why. In order to complete your makeover transformation you'll need to learn to not only listen to your instincts, but *trust* them.

It's often the whispers of your inner voice that allude to how *great* you can truly be.

~Lakeysha-Marie

CHAPTER FIFTEEN

Body Type Basics

You've probably guessed by now that dressing for your body type begins with a clear understanding of your body shape. It's how you learn to enhance your assets and incorporate balance for an attractive, streamlined silhouette.

Every one of us has physical attributes that make us unique; however, there are five general body types that you can use to determine your body shape: the ruler, inverted triangle, pear, hourglass, and apple. Read the descriptions below to discover which best defines your body shape, then follow the style tips provided to look your best. For the best assessment, observe yourself in the mirror wearing fitted apparel such as a swimsuit or undergarments. Remember, it's your *shape*, not your weight that determines your body type.

Ruler

Body Description:

- o Average to wide shoulders
- o Small to average bustline
- o Undefined waist
- o Straight hips and lower body

The Look:

Your body shape is a canvas for creating phenomenal looks! That build of yours will have no trouble looking great in a variety of skirts, dresses, and jeans. It goes without saying that your legs look great in sexy heels. To create the appearance of a curvier silhouette, select styles with volume and shape.

Inverted Triangle

Body Description:
- o Broad shoulders
- o Average to full bustline
- o Defined or undefined waist
- o Hips narrower than shoulders

The Look:

Your body type will shine in styles that soften your shoulder line and bring balance between your upper and lower body. Opt for tops and dresses in

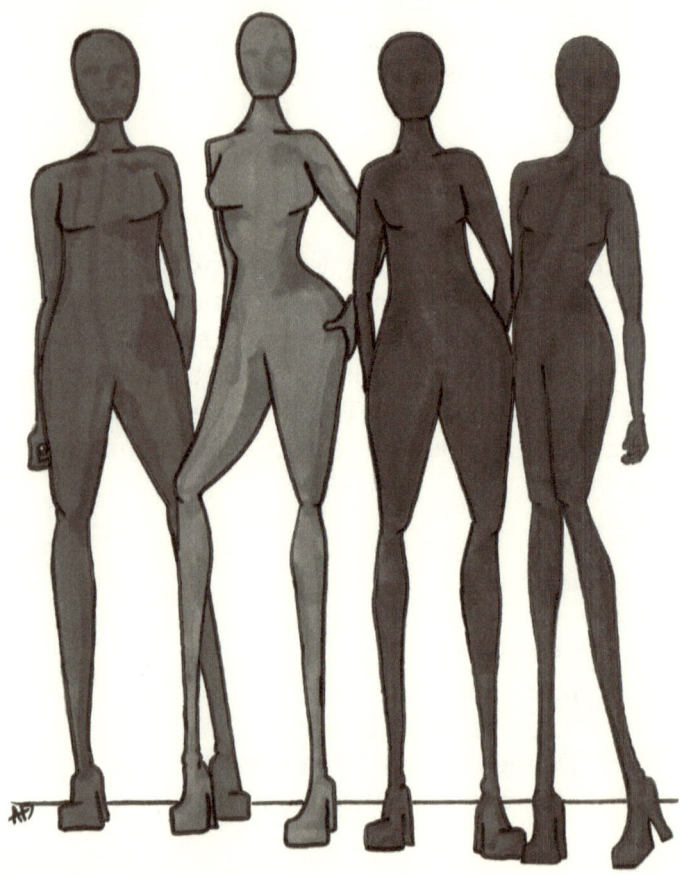

**Body types from left to right: apple, hourglass, pear, ruler
and inverted triangle.**

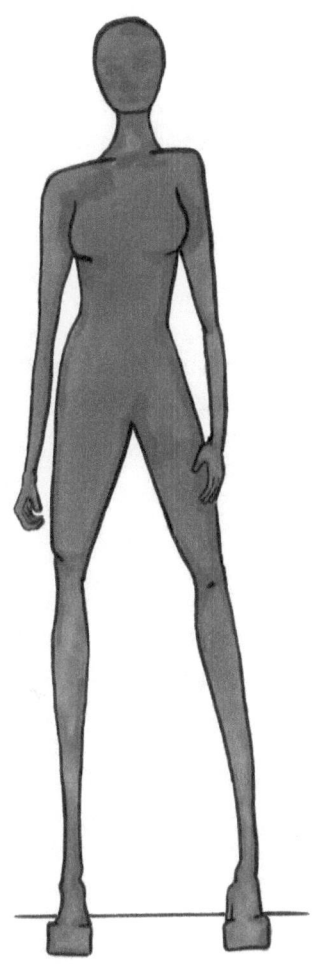

fabrics that drape as these materials will skim the body line and soften your silhouette. Open necklines such as scooped and v-necklines will offset your broad shoulders, as will raglan styles and shoulder slits on your sleeves. Adding volume through A-line skirts, bootcut jeans, and wide leg trousers will also create balance between your lower body and your shoulders.

Pear

Body Description:

- o Narrow or sloped shoulders
- o Small to average bustline
- o Defined waist
- o Full, curvy hips

The Look:

When selecting styles, your goal is to create a sexy, streamlined silhouette by balancing the width of your hips with your upper body. You can do this by selecting tops with beautiful details that draw the eye up and by selecting pant styles that minimize the fullness of your hips such as a wide leg and boot cut.

Hourglass

Body Description:

- o Average to full bustline

o   Defined waist
o   Equal hip and shoulder width

The Look:

You will want to put together a look that flatters your curves and accentuates the natural proportion of your body line. Do this by making your waist the focal point. Accent your curves with halter tops and dresses, wrap styles, belts, or the subtle flair of your favorite jean.

Apple

Body Description:

o   Average to wide shoulders
o   Average to full bustline
o   Full waist
o   Flat bottom
o   Slender legs

The Look:

Your most flattering look comes from styles that visually slim your torso and highlight your more slender lower body. Think raglan tops with a dark denim boot-cut jean, soft blouses paired with a tailored trouser, or a simple wrap dress with gorgeous heels to highlight your slender legs.

Keeping It in Proportion

Ever bought a cute pair of slacks labeled "P" only to take them home and discover the hem strangely hit three inches above your ankles? *Yes, this has happened to me…*

While it may seem obvious to some, it is easy to buy the wrong garment length if you do not understand height classifications. When shopping, you will find that fashion labels use three different categories for defining height: petite, average, and tall. It's important to know your height classification, as this will dictate the appropriate length and fit of the sleeve, pant leg, etc. These classifications can vary depending on the brand *and the woman,* but here is a useful starting point:

Petite (P): Five foot four and under

(163 centimeters and under)

Look for styles that are more tailored, not wide and baggy. This will balance the width of your body with your height.

Average: Five foot five to five foot eight

(165 centimeters to 173 centimeters)

Keep your height and width balanced by ensuring your sleeve and pant hems are the appropriate length. Pant hems that drag on the ground and sleeves that appear too short will detract from a polished appearance.

Tall (T): Five foot nine and above

(175 centimeters and above)

Styles that are long and wide, such as tops that hit below your hip and full-leg trousers, will complement your height and keep your look in proportion.

CHAPTER SIXTEEN

Fashion Essentials — Beautiful Basics

Having the basic fashion essentials makes it easier to coordinate a variety of looks, saving time and eliminating hassle.

Below is a brief list of timeless staples to help you put your best look forward.

The Suit. A tailored suit is more than a style for the office. Worn separately, the jacket looks great with jeans, worn over dresses, and paired with skirts. The trousers are just as versatile and look great with an assortment of tops.

The Shirt. Whether worn under a suit, or tied over a swimsuit, a button-down white shirt is a wardrobe staple. Select a style with seams and darts for shaping. This will give a figure-flattering silhouette.

The Skirt. A pencil skirt or an A-line skirt (flattering on fuller hips and thighs) in a clean,

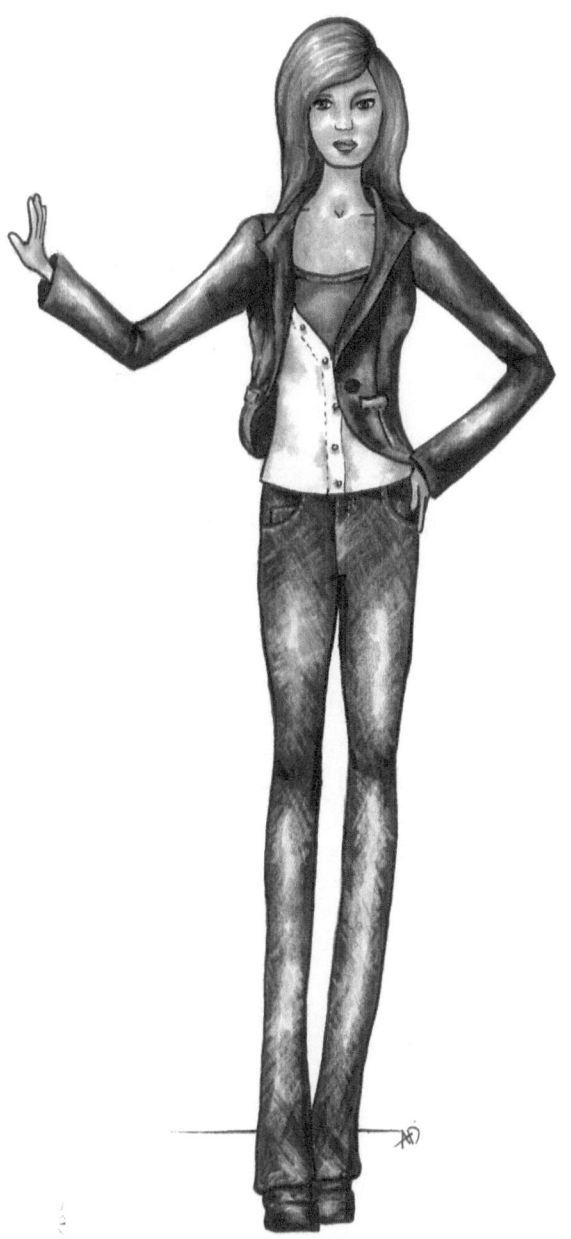

simple style makes a great transition piece from the office to a night out.

The Little Black Dress. This is *the* wardrobe staple. Dress it up or down for a look that's sexy and chic. It's what to wear when you have nothing to wear.

The Jean. Select either a slim-cut or boot-cut jean and buy it in a dark wash for maximum match-ability. Ensure this pair is long enough to wear with a low heel for a polished finish.

The Basics. Tees and tanks are great for layering as well as adding color and texture to your look. These affordable basics are great to stock up on.

Remember, the key to building a great wardrobe isn't limited to selecting designer one-of-a-kind pieces. Having a successful style means selecting items that can be worked into a variety of looks for maximum wearability. In the long run, it saves money and gives your wardrobe a longer life.

Here's to looking good.

CHAPTER SEVENTEEN

Selecting the Best Tees, Tops, and Blouses

Shopping can be daunting when it comes to the task of selecting tanks, tees, and blouses. As we peel layers off and on throughout the year, we are faced with the challenge of finding styles that not only highlight our sense of style but also look great on our body types.

The most common issues women face when shopping for tops are shoulder width, necklines, and exposing the shoulders and arms. In this chapter, I'll show you how to shop for tops to keep you looking oh so cool, without breaking a sweat.

Shoulder Width. Minimizing the width of a broader shoulder line can be done by selecting plain-front shirt styles without embellishments. For example, avoid tops with shoulder pads and puffed sleeves because they will make your shoulders appear wider than they really are. Also steer away from tops that have very thin straps...they have the same effect. Opt for tops with slightly wider straps to balance the width of your upper and lower body.

If you hail from the other end of the spectrum and have narrow or sloped shoulders, you will want to focus on the neckline of your summer tops to bring visual balance to your silhouette. Horizontal necklines, like boat necks and square necks, widen the appearance of your shoulders. Look for tops with details and trimming along the shoulder and sleeves to give the appearance of a wider shoulder line.

The Right Cut. Shopping for tops with a fuller bustline can present its own set of challenges, but sticking to the right styles can help you avoid common shopping pitfalls. One of the common tips circulating around the style realm is to wear a V-neck to minimize a full bustline, which in theory works, but how do you keep it appropriate?

The trick is to wear a *shallow* V-neckline or scooped-neckline top. The base of the V is higher and beautifully highlights the décolletage without exposing cleavage. Additionally, look for tank tops and camisoles that have wider straps. Thin spaghetti straps will not support your bustline and can cause the garment to shift down during wear. Finally, when you shop for tops, look for darts and seams that will give shape to your bust and torso. This ensures the top does not fit you at the bust and then hang in an unflattering, boxy shape.

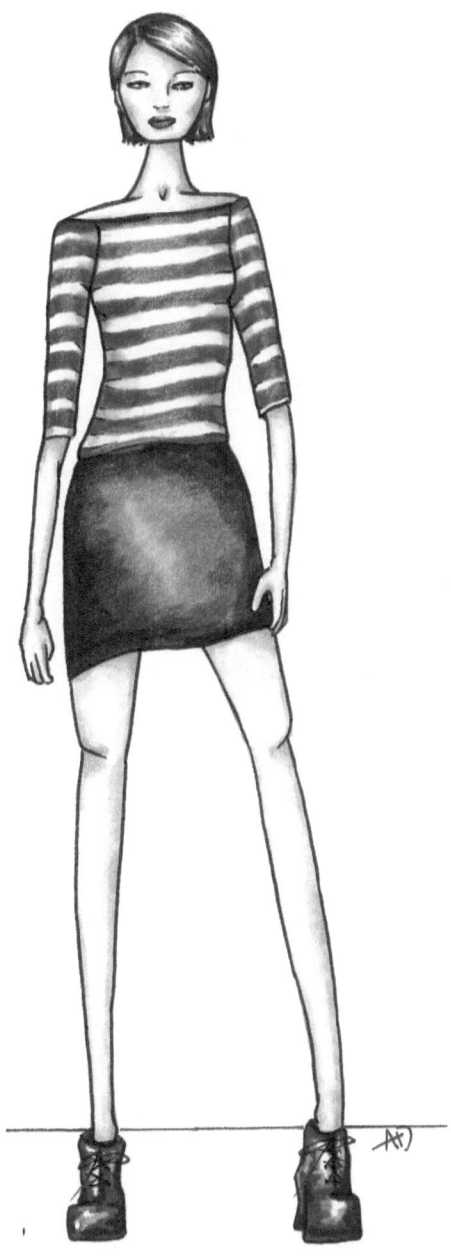

If you have a small bustline and would like to create more shape, look for tops with details along the bust such as pockets, ruching, gathers, and trims. They draw the eye up for a more shapely appearance.

Exposing Arms. Special occasions or warm weather mean shorter sleeves and exposed arms. For those who prefer to keep exposure of these limbs to a minimum, there are stylish options that will still keep you looking and feeling comfortably cool.

Three-quarter-length sleeves are great because they cover the part of the arm many of us have problems with, the upper arm, without restricting us to a full sleeve. A stylish shrug paired with a tank has the same effect. Another option is fluted sleeves; they drape nicely over arms creating a clean, flattering line.

CHAPTER EIGHTEEN

Chic White Shirt Basics

It's a good idea to invest in crisp white shirts — lots of them. The layer-ability factor of a chic white shirt makes it a classic item that can be worn every season.

Making the most of this garment boils down to cut, details, and balance. Here is a simple guide for selecting this stylish wardrobe staple and working it into your day-to-day looks.

The Right Fit. A simple white shirt in a tailored cut will create a solid foundation for quintessential style. The correct fit is a must for a clean appearance, so be sure to note the construction of the garment when shopping. The shoulder seams should align with the center of your shoulders, the collar should rest against the neck, and when buttoned the center front should lay flush with your body line without any pulling or gaping as a result of movement.

White blouses that are cut to drape have a looser fit but still require appropriate seaming to control the fabric for a flattering fit. Always try these styles on before buying to ensure the fabric drapes across your figure, giving a soft appearance that doesn't add bulk.

Devil in the Details. From ruffles along the neckline to wrap ties at the waist, there are plenty of stylicious details to give your basic white shirt a modern look. Remember, it's often the details that catch the eye and set the stage for showcasing your personal style.

Style Basics. We've addressed fit and designer details, now let's talk balance. Soft white blouses with a loose fit are best balanced with a structured pant, skirt, or jean.

For example, a soft satin blouse and a pencil skirt make the perfect pairing. The clean lines of a structured bottom visually balance out the volume of a softer blouse.

In contrast, a tailored white shirt will look great with just about anything. Why? The tailored cut reduces volume, making this an ideal style to layer under vests, sweaters, dresses, etc.

The Roll Back. Loosely rolled sleeves work well for day looks and are just the trick for accessorizing your basic white shirt with a statement cuff, bracelet, or timepiece. When pairing your white shirt with a sweater, jacket, or blazer, don't be

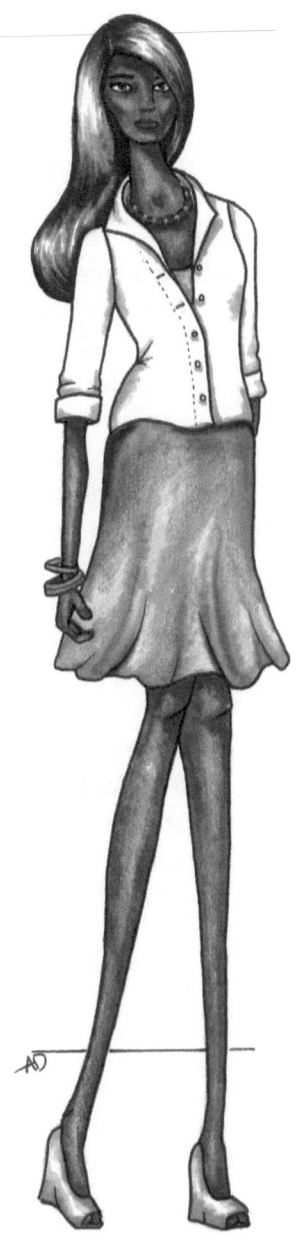

afraid to show a little cuff. It's an easy way to add a touch of style to a look and visually balance the white of your collar for a polished finish.

The Classic Combo. Pairing a crisp white shirt with denim is no big secret, but keep this look from becoming a boring basic by accessorizing appropriately. A stylish necklace will play up the V-neckline of a button-down shirt, and shape can be given to an untucked white shirt by adding a sash, textured belt, or leather tie.

Dress to Impress. I love the look of an immaculate white shirt paired with an A-line or pencil skirt, but adore it even more when paired with a dress. From wrap styles to sleeveless dresses, it's the perfect piece for bringing year-round wearability to your favorite dresses and providing an option for working evening pieces into a daytime look.

The versatility of a white shirt ranges from being the foundation of layered looks to stealing the show when paired with stellar accessories. Either way, be sure to get your hands on this must-have wardrobe staple and use it as a transitional piece for your wardrobe.

CHAPTER NINETEEN

The Advantages of Trousers

It has been said that the only constant in life is change, and thus began our never-ending struggle to prevent or accept it. I suppose working in the ever-evolving world of fashion has made it a little easier for me to accept. On countless occasions I have marveled at how dramatically a new outfit or a fresh hairstyle can alter a woman's appearance and skyrocket her level of confidence.

With that said, I have also learned that there is a homegrown comfort in classic elements that remain constant. It's a little like that love-worn hoodie stashed in the back of the closet that would probably horrify the makeover gurus of the reality TV world but makes the perfect companion on the rainiest of days.

Armed with this nostalgic style philosophy that some would deem reckless, I began flipping through the style reports only to discover that it was time to pay homage to an old favorite. A little more sophisticated than the hoodie, but a classic nonetheless. And might I add wearable?

An elegant, simple trouser evokes a sigh of relief from both fashion experts and novices alike. It provides a welcome shift from an industry exhausted by the cyclical trends of skinny jeans, harem pants, and tricky jumpsuits.

Perhaps the most appreciated element of this style is the wearability factor. Full figures benefit from the clean lines of the pant-leg as it smooths over full hips and thighs. At the same time, the fit-and-flare trousers accentuate lean hips and dramatically lengthen the leg line.

So, how do you wear this minimalist style and get the look of fuss-free glamour?

Balancing Act. Wearing an outfit that has volume on both the top and bottom will add width to your appearance. To avoid unwanted bulk, wide-leg trousers and flared pants are best balanced with sleek, fitted tops. Fail-safe options include tailored blouses, V-necks, wrap styles, and fitted tees. Stay cozy in the cooler months and minimize the fabric bulk by selecting fine-gauge knit tops to wear with this trouser style.

Vertical Height. The width of a wide-leg or flared pant can detract from your height. This is a common problem encountered by petite women. A simple solution is to visually balance the width of the pant leg with a pair of heels. Even a kitten heel

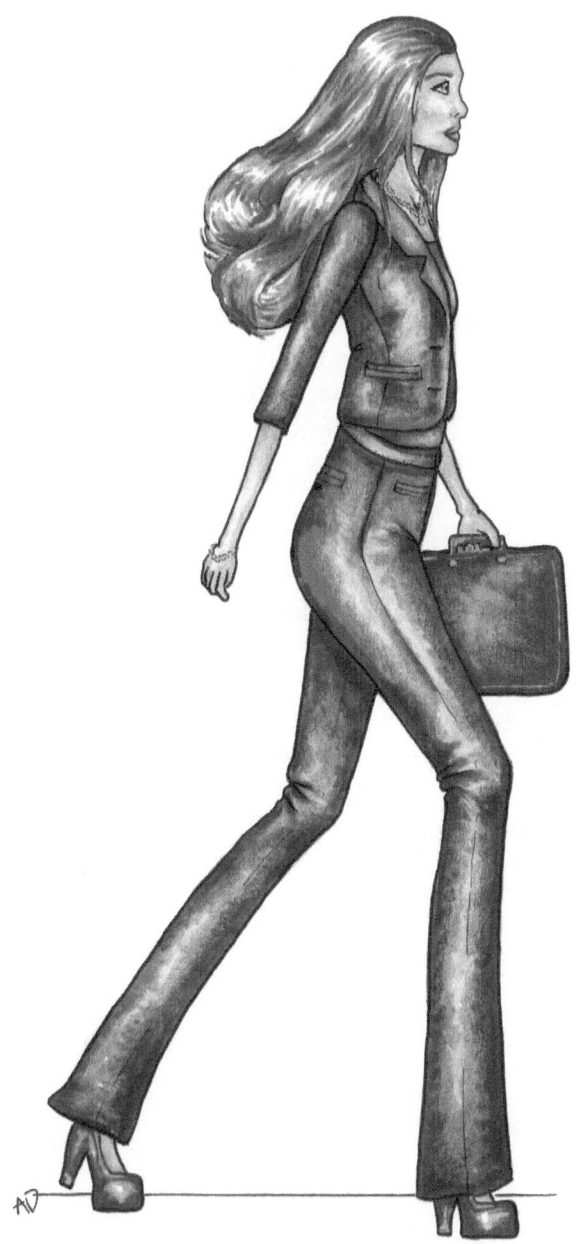

at minimum will lengthen the body line and keep hemlines from dragging along the ground and picking up debris.

Outerwear Details. Polish off chic trousers by pairing them with the right outerwear. We all love a cute puffer coat, but let's face it — arriving to a party looking sister to the Michelin man may impede your social progress. When the weather cools, top off stylish slacks with tailored A-line coats, fitted blazers, pea coats, and of course a cozy shearling jacket. From work to play, the clean lines of these designs bring a polished finish to almost any look.

Final thoughts? When it comes to wearing trousers, stay true to the style: basic, clean lines; good fabric drape; and a smart pair of heels.

And about that change thing? Embrace it. Always treat the world as your personal runway, remembering to update it with beautiful new collections along the way and never forgetting to keep a cozy hoodie for your rainy days.

CHAPTER TWENTY

It's a Woman's World: Figure-Flattering Skirts

L oved for their versatility and feminine sensibility, skirts are a wardrobe staple appreciated by all body types and fashion styles. To keep you well hemmed, here's the long and short of selecting the right skirt style.

Curvy. Show off the natural curves of your body in fabrics with good drape in flare, circle, or asymmetrical cuts. Styles such as straight skirts and A-lines help to minimize the appearance of full hips and bottom. Pencil skirts are flattering, but avoid versions of this style with hemlines that are very tapered (narrow at the hem), as this will visually widen your hips.

To avoid exaggerating the width of your hips, ensure your skirts have enough ease throughout the hip and thigh so the skirt does not cling or gather. Also, check for proper construction, such as darts and seaming, for the best shape and fit.

Slender. If you desire skirts that give more shape, look no further. A below-the-knee pencil skirt with a body-skimming fit that narrows at the knee will give the appearance of a curvier silhouette. Popular styles such as fluted, flare, and pleated skirts will also provide more shape to your silhouette.

For a shapelier bottom, look for skirts that skim along the hips and thigh and then flare out for an appealing silhouette. Remember to select cuts and fabrics that add volume and drape well, avoiding skirts that hang shapelessly from the body.

Tall and Petite. Balancing your height with your body shape is all about the hemlines. The best skirt lengths for petites to pick up this trend will be mid-calf to full-length skirts worn with heels. Longer hemlines require that you wear a heel to visually elongate your legs, giving your body a more balanced appearance.

The choice hemlines for tall women fall just below the knee or are full length. Fitted skirts worn just below the knee show off long legs while providing visual balance to the body. Play up long legs with a tiered skirt and heels for chic volume, or wear hemlines that stop just below the knee paired with your favorite boots.

Tops. As you shop for tops to wear with your longer skirts, opt for a fitted knit or tailored jacket to balance out the fullness of your skirt. Longer skirts are best worn with a V-neck, scooped neck,

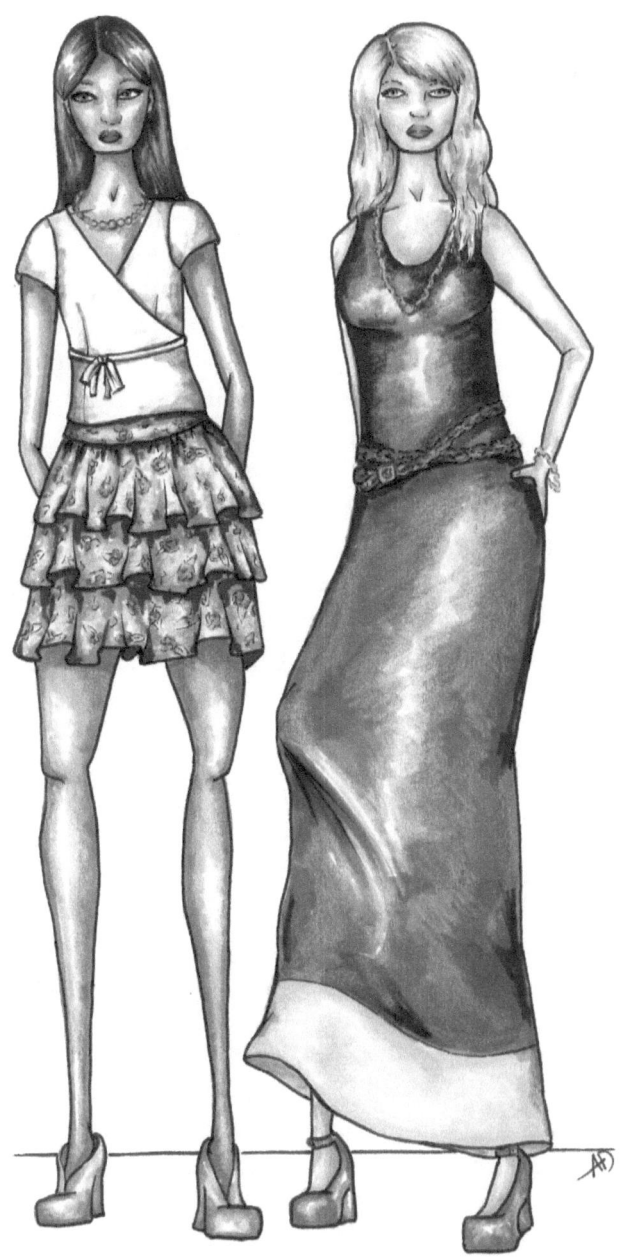

or other open necklines that will bring the eye up and create a strong vertical line.

Here's a snapshot of the top three skirt lengths:

The Mini. Look for this shorter, above-the-knee cut with a sophisticated take on styling. Sweet flounce miniskirts, tiered layers, and ruffle details are a few of the key miniskirt styles that will continue to make fashion edits season after season. The softer color palettes popular in spring will dress up this skirt style and makes it a workable option for blending into an existing wardrobe. Tulip style and high-waist miniskirts are also fashionable options for creating a leggier look. For a dressier option, focus on fabric and style details. Pretty rosettes, sheer layers, and fabrics that drape well can make an everyday look into something truly special.

The Midi. No stranger to the fashion magazines, the midi skirt is continually updated with versatile colors and patterns. For many this skirt hybrid represents the perfect balance between a chic miniskirt and a fashionable maxi skirt. The hem of this skirt style typically hits the mid calf, providing more coverage than a miniskirt, but still allowing the wearer to show a little more leg than possible with a maxi skirt. Generally, you can find this ladylike style in floral prints, classic A-line shapes, and colorful solids. Pair with a sexy blouse to keep this skirt from looking too prim, but still very proper. Play up the feminine mood of this skirt style with chiffon blouses, asymmetric tops, or a structured high heel.

The Maxi. A dominant year-round favorite, the maxi-length skirt proves that skin isn't always in when it comes to looking gorgeous. The full length of a maxi skirt can be casually paired with a knit tank and boots or dressed up with a pair of heels and accessories that shimmer for a beautiful, fuss-free evening look. I love the look of this skirt in fascinating tribal prints, subtle sheers, modern bubble hems, and metallic threads for a chic sheen to polish off a day or night look. A looser-cut maxi skirt will flow better over curves, while the more structured maxi-skirt styles are great for emphasizing curves and visually adding height. Stack on the style by pairing maxi skirts with the season's sculpted wedge heels.

As always, when shopping for your favorite skirt styles, remember to pay close attention to cut and fabric drape to ensure the best fit and look for your body type.

CHAPTER TWENTY-ONE

Five Denim Looks to Wear Now

Our favorite weekend fallback is *hot*, always. Denim continually lights up the retail racks, showcasing patches, distressed treatments, and enough cuts to have every fashionista singing the blues.

Explore a softer side of denim by mixing floral prints with distressed denims for a fresh, feminine look or rock edgy denim styles with leather accessories and denim handbags.

The versatility of designs that major fashion houses provide makes denim an easy addition to both day and night looks. Whether paired with smart trainers or peep-toe heels, this street-chic trend is a must for updating your look.

Seeking a bit of style inspiration? Here are five denim looks that you can wear anytime:

1. Fun screen-printed tees and distressed denim go hand in hand. Denim can be purchased pre-distressed or simply create your own signature style with scissors and your favorite jean.

2. Gorgeous frocks take on an edgy-sweet flavor when topped off with a denim jacket. For a figure-flattering fit, select jackets that have plenty of seams and darts for shaping.

3. Shiny denim jeans with heels are perfect for grooving the night away. Look for this finish in dark blue hues and intense black denim.

4. Keep denim daytime chic by pairing your dark-wash denims with a tailored blouse and smart pumps. To ensure a polished appearance, jeans must be hemmed long enough to wear with heels.

5. Denim skirts look fantastic with embellished flats or flirty wedges. Elongate your leg line by pairing a knee-length denim skirt with wedges, boots, or a heel. In contrast, denim minis are best balanced with flats.

Keep in mind that this is merely a starting point—denim is a material every woman can truly make her own. With its versatility, our favorite throwback to comfort has clearly secured an eternal spot in our wardrobe as a stylish staple.

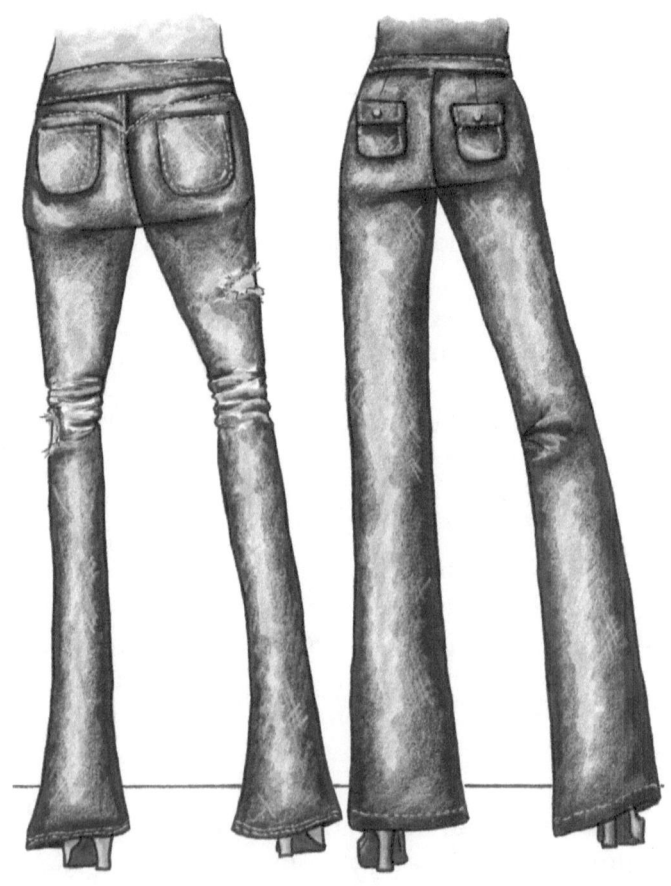

Denim silhouettes from left to right: bootcut, wide leg, straight leg, and skinny.

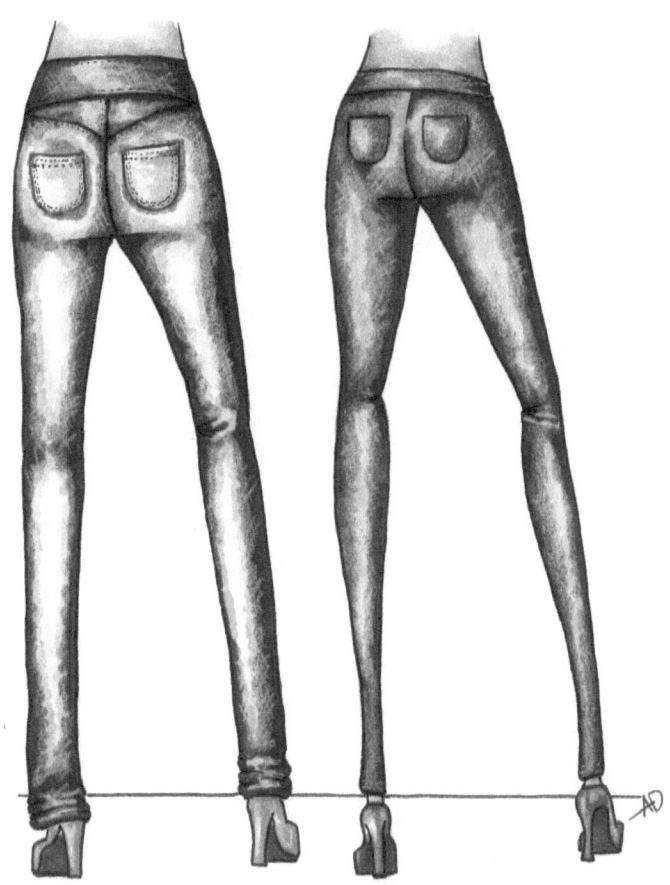

CHAPTER TWENTY-TWO

The Little Black Dress

The little black dress is frequently hailed as one of the most important pieces of a woman's wardrobe; and with good reason. It's a garment that can take her seamlessly to the boardroom layered under a polished blazer, into an unforgettable evening look when paired with gorgeous accessories and heels. Oh, and let's not forget the weekend chic of a belted LBD under a cozy cardigan with soft leather boots. With so many ways to wear it, your only real challenge will be finding the right one to flatter your shape. So let's get started!

Ruler. Your athletic body shape can easily transition between dress styles and you may find that your biggest hurdle is visually adding curves or softening your athletic look. If fitted styles that highlight your bodyline are your preference LBDs with an asymmetric shoulder line, tapered pencil skirt or sleek tulip hem is the perfect segue to breath taking style.

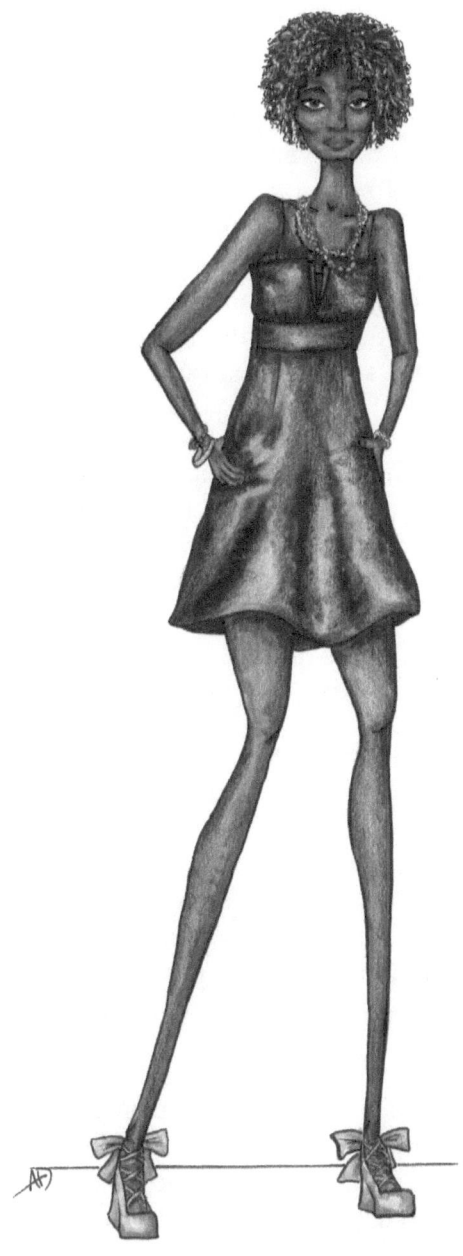

Add curves with feminine details such as dramatic cowls, waist defining peplums, sexy ruching and voluminous gathers.

Pear. The curves of your lower body look stunning in dresses that have either an A-line skirt or a straight skirt. Why? These styles skim over curvy hips and thighs creating a balanced and beautiful hemline. Remember, the goal is not to hide your curves; it's to balance them. Highlight your upper body in a dress with a strapless, halter or spaghetti strap bodice.

Inverted Triangle. The best little black dress for your shape is a style that softens your shoulder line while balancing the curves of your upper body with your slender lower body. This can be stylishly accomplished with v- necklines dresses that drape, fit and flare dresses, A-line dresses, wrap styles and of course the classic sheath.

Hourglass. Keep your LBD style effortless by making your waist the focal point of your silhouette. This can be achieved with belted dresses, wrap styles and clever side panels that draw the eye in. Fitted styles best show off your shape however if you prefer a flowing style, accessorize your LDB with a belt to ensure your curves do not disappear beneath the volume of the fabric.

Apple. Flaunt your beautiful shape by selecting a LBD that highlights your slender arms and legs. Think fluid tunic styles that hit the knee, silk blouson dresses, and asymmetric cuts that will flatter your arms. If you tend to carry extra weight around your middle like most apples, this can be easily balanced with a scoop or V neckline that will visually bring the eye up. While empire line dresses are a classic choice for this body shape, keep your LBD modern by pairing this silhouette with a flattering belt worn just below the bust.

CHAPTER TWENTY-THREE

Seasonal Dress Fundamentals

Whether it's spring or fall, a time comes for us to switch out our interim wardrobes with refreshing apparel styles, and few things epitomize the shift in seasons like a beautiful eye-catching dress.

Step into any store and you will see a plethora of dresses decorating the racks, but the act of choosing the perfect dress may prove to be a trickier endeavor. Picking the right style begins with knowing the trends, understanding your body type, and of course, throwing in that added spark that we call personality.

Style Factors. For women who traditionally find themselves limited when it comes to shopping the seasonal trends, selecting a new dress may now come a little easier. Dresses are being limited less and less to a specific color trend or print, providing more option for those wanting to spruce up their look.

If you prefer to pick up on the rainbow of colors infused into the key looks of the season, color options traditionally range from refreshing pastels of spring to the crisp, cool whites and quenching sorbets in the summer to the rich browns and luscious wine hues of autumn/winter.

Soft floral prints continually resurface as a popular seasonal staple, but don't be afraid to try this print depicted in intensely bright colors that allude to the longer days of summer.

Ever present in warm weather are tribal-inspired prints with palettes that range from neutral to bright. These styles available in varying lengths from maxi to mini dresses designed to either highlight or comfortably conceal.

Picking the Right Silhouette. As always, a solid understanding of your body shape is essential for selecting a flattering spring dress. A shapeless shift rarely does anyone any good, no matter what the body type is. Shop with the features you would like to enhance in mind. This will allow you to mentally weed out styles that do not fit your ideal.

If you have a fuller lower body, select a dress in a cut that is fitted throughout the upper body and then gradually widens as it falls toward the hem. Defined waists on all body shapes look great in belted or wrap-style dresses.

Not so keen on showing off your arms? Leave the jacket in the closet and opt instead for a dress with beautiful kimono-style or fluted sleeves. For those looking to add shape to their silhouette, look for dresses that have an A-line shape to the skirt or subtle tiered layering in a flattering print.

Add Some Personality. In order to look and feel fabulous in a new spring dress, it has to suit your taste and personality. Look for accents in the dress that incorporate elements reflective of you. For example, those who gravitate toward minimalism would radiate in a dress in a classic color with clean, strong lines.

In contrast, those with a romantic style would be better suited in a dress enhanced by ruffles and bow details. Find the details that resonate with your inner style diva and so that you can truly make the perfect dress you discover your own.

CHAPTER TWENTY-FOUR

Evening and Holiday Style

Whether you are a budding socialite, have a special night out planned, or have simply been sucked into one of the many holiday seasons, when it comes to parties, family get-togethers, and festive events with friends, you'll want to always look your best.

Initially this all sounds exciting, but unless you have the time and budget to buy a dress for every occasion, you will need a creative twist to keep your nighttime look fresh and full of style. From the beauty counter to the fitting room, I've compiled a list of the style tricks for pulling off seamless evening style.

A Bold Belt. Give your dress a new style lift with either an embellished or color-rich belt worn at the waist. Bold color will add a modern twist, while a jeweled or metallic belt will contribute to a luxe look. An ideal belt for this look is a waist cincher. Made to be worn at the waist, these styles offer

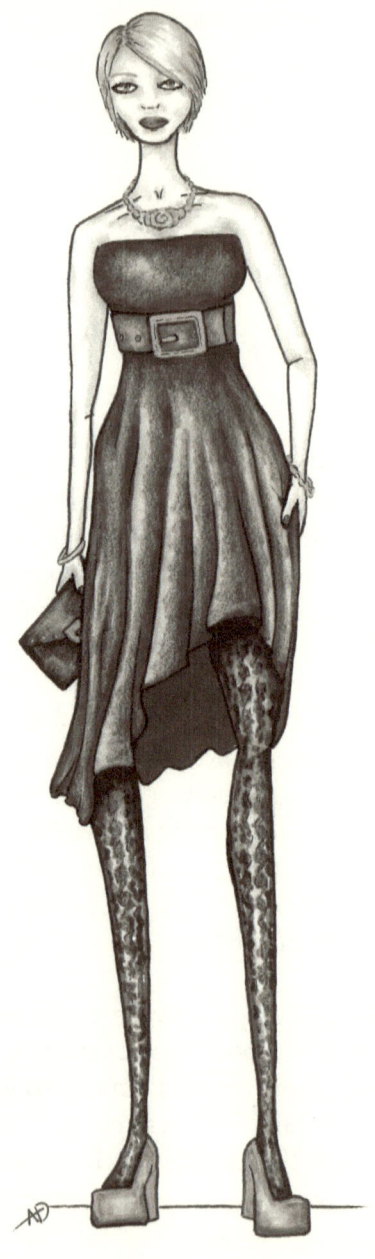

simple front closure along with an elasticized back for additional comfort.

Patterned Legwear. Few things are certain in life, but one thing guaranteed is that nude and black sheer tights are guaranteed to make a cameo at every venue and party. Add a splash of style and differentiate your look from the crowd by pairing your party dress with patterned hosiery. From a subtle metallic hose that adds sheen to sophisticated herringbone patterns, it's a fantastic way to dress up legs and add pop to your evening look.

Layer Your Look. Adding a layer will quickly revamp an old dress. Great layering options include tailored blazers, capelets, shrugs, and structured leather jackets. Depending on the cut and style of your dress, layers can seamlessly blend into your look or become a fashionable focal point.

Take Center Stage. A red-carpet favorite, statement necklaces are just the trick for refreshing an LBD (little black dress) or simple dress. This accessory is perfectly paired with open necklines, strapless styles, and plunging V-necks. When wearing a statement piece, be sure to keep the rest of your accessories minimal for a balanced look.

Shine On. Revamp your favorite frock with heels, clutches, and accessories that sparkle. Shoes with metallic finishes and bedazzled handbags instantly refresh your look and give new life to your evening dress.

CHAPTER TWENTY-FIVE

The Skinny on Belts

By now, many of you have made your style wish list and have checked it twice. But if you are missing this go-to accessory, you may want to re-access your style registry. Wrap your wardrobe collections with the smooth contours of a slender belt.

It's a versatile accessory that easily transitions from day to night, and I've got the skinny on how to wear the look!

Get the Party Started. Bejeweled and embellished skinny belts will bring definition to your party look, adding an unexpected dazzle as they catch the light. A gold leather skinny is a solid holiday staple, but don't be afraid to step outside the box.

Thin velvet belts are perfect for a textural contrast against silks, satins, and sheer styles. A basic dress can quickly transition into a look of seemingly

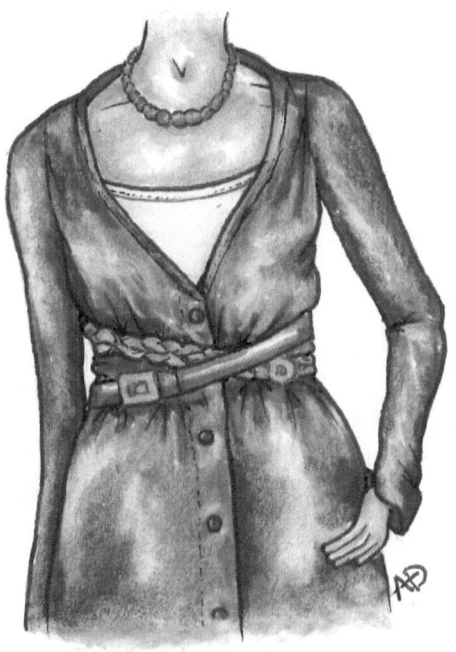

effortless glamour when accessorized with a skinny that has crystals, rhinestones, sequins, or any other metallic finish.

Work It. Skinny belts will bring a stylish infusion to any work wardrobe. A streamlined leather skinny looks great worn over blouses, fitted knit tops, and tailored jackets. The latter is a favorite runway look that can be realistically and easily incorporated into real day. Wear a tailored jacket over a thin blouse and then belt your skinny at your natural waist. The clean lines of the tailored jacket will keep your upper body structured, and the belt will soften the look by defining the waist for a feminine silhouette.

The same skinny belt can also be worn with work trousers, skirts, and day dresses. Due to their size, skinny belts are perfect for adding a balanced splash of color to workwear neutrals. Red and orange leathers contrast beautifully against blacks and browns, while purple, pink, and blue leathers accent cool grays for a stylish twist. Who knew getting ready for work could be so fun?

Day to Day. A casual skinny can be aptly paired with our laidback layers of winter. Think longer knit tees, fitted sweaters, and grandpa cardigans. It can even be worn to bring shape and structure to a bulkier knit. We also love the modern update that a skinny will bring to a winter coat. By swapping out the original belt for a single or double skinny, you can quickly refresh an old winter coat for a chic winter look.

Placement. Skinny belts can be worn at the natural waist, slung low over the hips or just below the bustline. Wearing a belt just below the bust will create a solid line that will immediately draw the eye. Keep your look interesting by selecting a skinny belt that has either color or texture. Think distressed leathers, textured crocs, and sleek patents. Sweet details such as bows and velvets work well for this placement.

When wearing a skinny belt at the natural waist or hips, a fun way to update this look is to double up on the belts. Two skinny belts worn together will add a fashionable air that you just don't get from wearing a single, standard belt. This style also looks stunning with dresses that drape and flow with the movement of the body. Doubling up on the skinny will also bring proportion to a fuller silhouette. A single skinny may emphasize a fuller figure, while doubling the skinny or opting for a medium-width belt will bring balance to the silhouette.

CHAPTER TWENTY-SIX

The Importance of Handbags

One of my favorite ways to update a wardrobe and pick up the season's trends is with a brand-new handbag. A well selected addition can update your look from everyday to exceptional with a simple swap of a tote.

Tassel handbags, exotic fabrics, and bursts of bright, bold colors also contribute to the stylish mix of handbag styles available to eager fashionistas season after season.

Those with a more casual take on style can also happily indulge in the comfortable handbags constructed from canvas, linen, and cotton materials. With that said, identifying the style is only half the battle and selecting the correct purse to flatter your shape isn't always easy. Let's review the best styles for balancing your look with a selection of trendy totes.

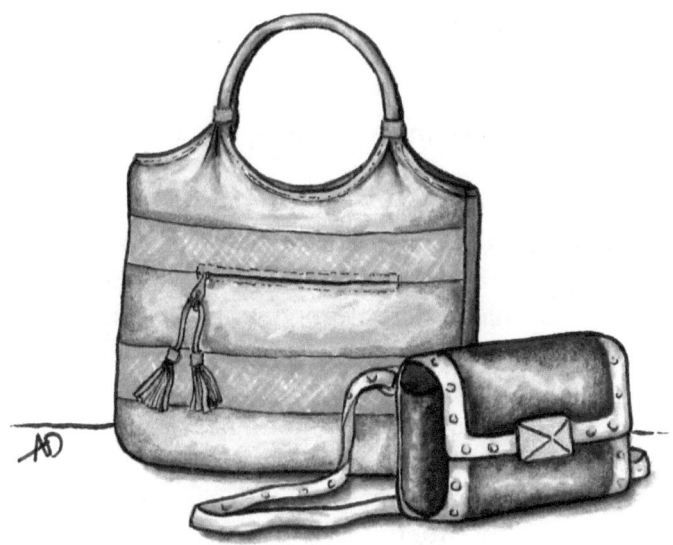

A common challenge for tall women is finding a cute handbag that looks good against a longer body frame. What do I suggest? Think size and volume to balance out a lengthy body line. Slouchy bags, totes, clutches, and oversize styles are top picks for bringing visual balance to a woman of height.

At the other end of the spectrum, large bags will dwarf a petite frame. Small- to medium-size handbags work best for this height. Focus on embellishment and detail instead of volume and length when selecting a handbag to accent your look.

If your aim is to balance out the curves of your silhouette, the length of your handbag strap will play a vital role in determining which handbag style will work best for you. For example, a pear-shaped woman has an average upper body, but tends to carry more weight along her hips and thighs. To detract from a fuller lower body and highlight a leaner upper body, select a handbag worn on the shoulder with shorter straps. This will bring the eye up and balance the curves throughout the length of the body line.

If the opposite holds true for you and you tend to carry your weight along your upper body, opt instead for a bag with a longer strap that hits the waist. Handbags without shoulder straps such as clutches and handheld totes are other fashionable options.

Wondering which purse styles work best for all-over curves? This silhouette is best balanced by structured handbags and sturdy totes. Avoid handbags constructed from flimsy fabrics and teeny prints as these can look disproportionate against a fuller silhouette.

With so much arm candy to choose from, it's important to select a bag that not only accents your clothing but also flatters your body shape. Shop wisely.

CHAPTER TWENTY-SEVEN

Selecting Your Best Colors

From sultry wines to sophisticated blues, it's no surprise that color is one of the most important elements of a woman's wardrobe and almost critical when it comes to making the best impression. Choosing the right shade can awaken tired skin and even take years off our appearance. Colors have the power to impact the way we look and feel, affecting our moods and even those around us.

But how do we determine which colors work best for us? It may not be as tricky as you think. The colors we see in clothing and cosmetics fall into one of two categories: blue-based colors and yellow-based colors. Blue-based colors look best on cool skin tones while yellow-based colors look best on warm skin tones.

What Is My Skin Tone? The best way to determine if your skin tone is cool or warm is to look at your skin in natural daylight against a white surface. Easiest way? Wrap a white towel around your hair and another around your body, leaving your

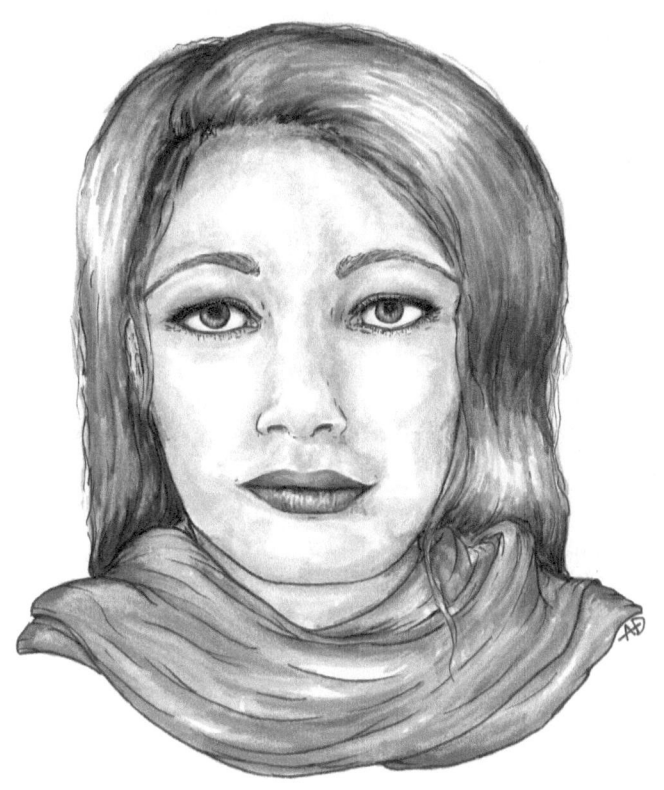

shoulders and face exposed. When under natural daylight (i.e., the light coming in through a window), look at the undertone of your skin in your reflection. Cool skin tones can be rosy, olive, or blue-black while warm skin tones are more golden or peachy.

Helpful Hints. Women with cool skin tones characteristically have eye colors such as deep brown, gray, gray-blue, blue, hazel (brown and green), and light brown. Natural hair colors include raven black, medium to dark brown, platinum blonde, ash blonde, salt and pepper, cool gray, and crisp white.

Women with warm skin tones characteristically have eye colors that are more golden in hue such as rich dark brown, golden brown, moss green, soft blue, and warm hazel (brown and green with gold). Natural hair colors include golden brown, chestnut, golden blonde, strawberry blonde, red, auburn, and golden gray.

Choosing the Right Colors. Cool skin tones look radiant in rich vibrant colors and cool pastels. Some of your best colors include royal blue, emerald green, ruby red, silver, rich plum, frosty pinks, and aqua blues.

Warm skin tones look wonderful in warm earthy colors. Some of your best colors include bronze, coral red, olive green, soft ivory, mocha, cinnamon, rich pumpkin, and gold.

Making It Work. The next time you are out

shopping, check the color along with the price tag. Have a look at your reflection and ask yourself...

- o Does it bring out my eyes?
- o Does it add a warm glow to my skin?
- o Do I look refreshed?

And lastly, don't forget to experiment with new colors. It's the only way to find your winning combination.

CHAPTER TWENTY-EIGHT

How to Work Color into Your Look

Pastel hues and classic colors are traditional palettes, but vivid hues bring a welcome energy to many a wardrobe. Lush orange, muted tangerine sorbet, lemon yellow, and splashes of grapefruit red all contribute to the revitalizing energy that is style.

For many stylists, introducing someone to a new color is often like teaching a bird to fly. They strategically wait until the unsuspecting chick is on the edge and then they push her.

While this approach has been proven successful in the wild, when it comes to shopping for a new color a different approach is required. Unlike flying, choosing color is often a personal expression, not a requirement. If you don't feel a connection or meaning to a color then it just won't fly. To keep you in harmony with both your inner being and your wardrobe, I offer simple suggestions for incorporating bold color into your look.

If slow and easy is your approach, swap out your black, gray, and navy apparel for a lighter neutral shade. Classic white, khaki, and cream are neutrals that will take you throughout the year. These neutral hues will also complement jewel-colored hues, as seen with the sophisticated mix of khaki and orange.

Purchasing outerwear apparel in vivid colors can do wonders to update your look and extend the lives of your favorite items. The heavy black overcoats of winter can be swapped out for lightweight jackets and coats in hues of white, green, blue, and red.

Alternatively, transition a winter jacket or trench into the cooler evenings of spring by updating with a vibrant scarf or swapping out the original belt with a bolder color option for a stylish spring statement. A camel trench coat paired with a red belt will quickly bring the coat up to date, or try the stylish twist of a black jacket paired with a deep purple belt.

CHAPTER TWENTY-NINE

Finding Neutral Ground

The neutral color palettes available offer many a demure alternative to bright color trends. Subtle champagnes, blush hues, whites, and taupe are just a few of neutral shades prevalent on the runways.

However, as sophisticated as these colors may seem, it's easy to appear washed out when neutral color palettes are not appropriately paired. The key to taking these shades from runway to real day is texture, color, and contrast.

Work the Surface. From a traditional standpoint, neutral colors do exactly what their name implies. This family of understated hues is used to bring balance to vibrant and highly saturated colors. As a result they often get the reputation of being the wallflowers of the fashion party and even considered at times to be boring — *gasp!* With that said, there are several ways to breathe life into your neutrals to create an eye-catching color combination.

Avoid the drab and boring look of neutrals by bringing the surface of the material to life with a textured fabric. Look for neutrals that have a slight sheen or select styles that use threads with luster to give visual interest to everyday neutral colors. Mixing and matching neutral textures that have a ruched surface, ruffles, silk, and sheer fabrics will also aid in giving more depth and intrigue to your look.

Designer embellishments such as stitched-down cream-colored pearls, 3-D neutral-toned flowers, and neutral styles with unfinished edges will bring a fashionable twist to an otherwise ordinary garment.

Contrasting Trims. Working in contrasting accessories and trims is another way to prevent looking washed out when wearing neutral shades. An excellent example of this is the classic trench coat. It is rare to see a neutral trench coat or jacket that has not been finished with contrasting trims. It's the tortoiseshell buttons, dark piping along the lapel, or even a simple black plastic buckle that adds a stylish finish to an otherwise basic jacket.

The same applies to piecing items together for a neutral-based outfit. Neutral dresses look great with a dark contrasting belt and heels. Neutral blouses are the perfect backdrop for accenting a darker accessory piece, and it goes without saying that neutral trousers and skirts really pop when paired with a contrasting shoe.

Blend in Color. Wake up your neutral items by blending a richer color hue into your look. However popular nudes may be, for most women beige as a standalone color is not flattering, but mix it with a deep chocolate brown or a crisp, clean white with metallic accessories and suddenly you have my attention. Neutrals are made to be mixed with other colors and can be comfortably worn with pinks, blues, and greens.

The same result can also be achieved through colorful accessories found in intense purples, reds, and other citrus hues. In contrast, if the focal point of an outfit is a bright color, use neutral colors to bring balance to the look and offset the color intensity.

CHAPTER THIRTY

The Upside to Blue

A sea of blue in the form of smart suits, flowing gowns, and dramatic accessories is just the thing to keep this color looking anything but under the weather.

The Right Shade. Infusing the right shade of blue into your apparel or accessories has the power to brighten the eyes and give radiance to a worn complexion. Warm skin tones and olive complexions are best complemented with turquoise hues and vibrant teals. On the other end of the spectrum, cobalt, navy, and purple-based blues are just the trick for cool skin tones. For high impact style, look for your favorite hue of blue in fashion items that will be worn near the face for optimal results. Think lightweight scarves, blouses, and hats for an intense pop of color that is right on point.

Colorful Coordinates. Admittedly, when it comes to match-ability, black always steals the spotlight in the world of fashion. Black makes us looks slim.

Black matches everything. It lets people know not to mess with us.

Blue typically plays second fiddle to black as a classic shade, but don't be surprised to learn it can be matched with nearly every color. What you pair your blue with will depend heavily on your personality and your mood. Traditional blues such as navy and periwinkle look great when combined with neutrals such as khaki, white, and tan. Teals and Tahitian blues invite a more tropical and exotic feel when paired with purples, soft pinks, and emerald greens.

For those with the "go bold or go home" mind-set, take a cue and fearlessly combine intense royal blue with fuchsia, orange, or electric green for a color explosion worthy of a *Vogue* fashion edit.

Royal Treatments. Whether it's a cocktail ring, handbag, or peep-toe pump, accessory lovers will find it available in a flattering deep sea hue. These proportional pieces of style candy are as versatile as they are beautiful, but to really set off your blues, pair them with a simple look.

Blue accents create an ideal contrast when worn with everyday neutral shades. Add a splash of color to white by incorporating a vibrant blue handbag or turquoise belt. Monochrome evening looks in black can be quickly brought up to date by pairing with a royal-blue heel or navy satin flats. And if sapphire truly symbolizes mental clarity and perception, then consider me focused. This gemstone takes front and center as an elegant way to pick up the tranquil side of fashion.

Ladies, plan your cocktail looks accordingly.

CHAPTER THIRTY-ONE

Metallics — Born to Shine, Baby

L ooking for a bit of style and luxury? Spoil yourself *and* your wardrobe by indulging in the eye-catching glamour of gold metallic accents.

If shimmery fabrics, decadently embellished accessories, and polished glinty heels melt your heart to gold, then you will undoubtedly want to incorporate this element into your A-list looks. The key to successfully wearing this glamorous hue is to ensure that each gold piece flows evenly with the rest of the outfit and does not overpower. To help keep your look in check, read on as I share smart style secrets for accessorizing with gold.

Color Combinations. Gold is a color that when worn standalone as a dress makes a serious style statement. However, if you are looking to blend and mix your gold with additional colors, here are a few combinations you may want to try. Intense black velvet hues create an ideal canvas for gold appliqués, threading, and brocades. I also love the

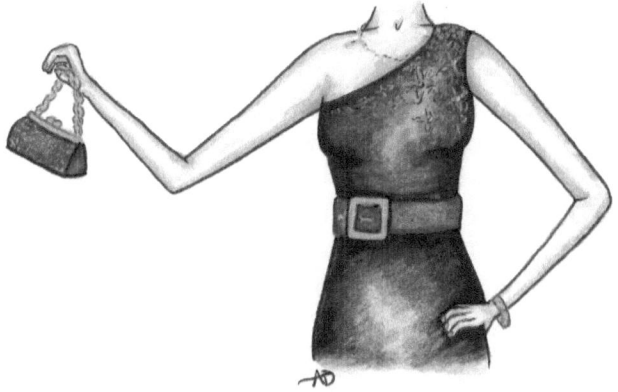

look of gold when paired with rich wine reds, earthy greens, crisp whites, clear blues, and of course, deep chocolate browns.

Day Glow. Soft gold leathers paired with denim will also work to add a healthy dose of glam to an otherwise basic day look. Hobo-inspired metallic day bags and gold ballet flats are stylish additions for running around town. A soft matte pump in gold also adds a touch of sophisticated sheen when worn with skirts, trousers, and day dresses.

Evening Glamour. This opulent metallic shade may be just the remedy for glamming up an evening look, but as always balance is key. The golden rule for flawlessly incorporating this color into jewelry and apparel is to not overdo it. Whether you wear a lean, straight-leg gold trouser or a statement necklace with the Midas touch, choose your focal point and keep the rest of your look simple. This will give your evening look a sophisticated serving of bling, without the " I just robbed a treasure chest" effect.

Working It In. For those looking for a quick update to a current wardrobe, work this look in with solid gold cuffs, belt buckles, and gold leather accessories. My favorites include gold leather evening clutches, skinny belts, and gold-beaded handbags that radiate style.

Including gold accents is a great way to update and refresh your look any season. Whether it's a chunky bracelet paired with a flirty frock or metallic pumps to dress up your favorite denims, remember to wear your gold strategically for well-balanced bling.

Shine on, Golden Girls. Shine on.

CHAPTER THIRTY-TWO

Animal Prints: A Guide to Walking on the Wild Side

Take a walk on the wild side by swapping out the traditional dark brown and tan leopard print for a more exotic color palette. Think striking leopard prints in deep blue and gray hues prowl the fabric and accessory boards while playful giraffe prints infused with golden accents gracefully walk down retail aisles.

If your goal is to take this look from runway to real day, you will need to have the appropriate color pairing for your animal prints.

Animal Instinct. Pairing an animal print with a tonal neutral such as tan, white, gray, brown, or black is a simple way to keep your animal prints tame. Blue animal prints are beautifully accented with cool gray apparel and accessories and I love the look of a pink-hued animal print paired with the crisp whites of the season. For those who prefer the tried-and-true options, zebra will always match black and tan will soften the look of a brown leopard or cheetah print.

will always match black and tan will soften the look of a brown leopard or cheetah print.

Lead the Pack. A splash of animal print is an ideal method of adding a healthy dose of style to your day looks. For a more casual option, pair your animal print with denim. Try matching an animal top with jeans and flats, or topping off an animal-print dress with a denim jacket. An animal-print scarf worn with the basic tees and tanks is also a safe way to minimally work this trend into your wardrobe for maximum style.

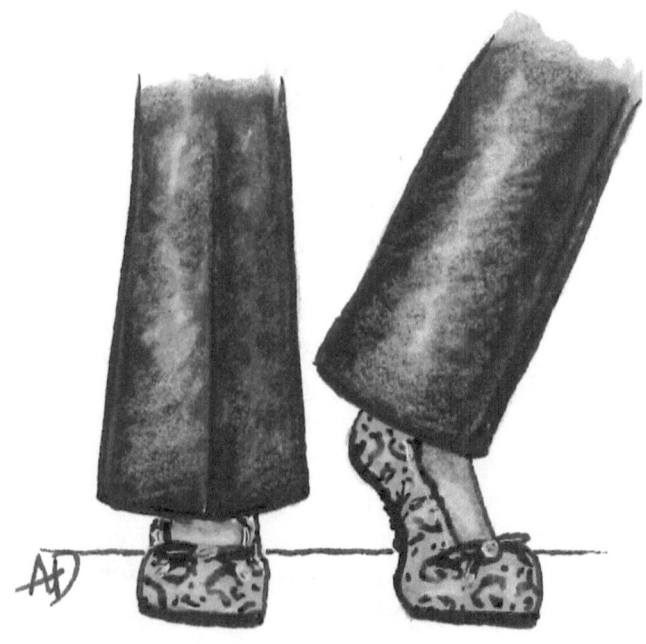

Style Prowess. Animal-print accessories are designed to catch the eye, making them an ideal accompaniment to evening looks. For maximum impact, animal-print accessories should be worn with solid colors.

A sleek purple snakeskin clutch will quickly update a little black dress and a gray leopard-print peep-toe is just the remedy for setting off a pair of charcoal trousers. Combining your animal prints with leather will give an edgy contrast to your look or alternatively, animal prints in sheer fabrics will add a feminine flair to your outfit.

CHAPTER THIRTY-THREE

How to Wear Lace

Lingerie. Doilies. Elizabethan collars. Excusing the latter, all common images that come to mind when referencing lace.

As a fashion stylist, I have to admit that lace often gets a bad rap as a fabric of extremes. Faced with the bleak propaganda of being overtly racy or crisp and stuffy, it's often whisked away to the clearance rack long before the season has ended.

However, with a little encouragement, lace can be incorporated into seamless styles and intricate accents that exude grown-up sexy. With that said, lace is a sensitive fabric that should be worn strategically.

Stay Focused. Select one lace garment to be the focal point of the outfit and keep the rest of your look basic. In doing so you will balance the lace and ensure you don't arrive looking like a new pair of drapes.

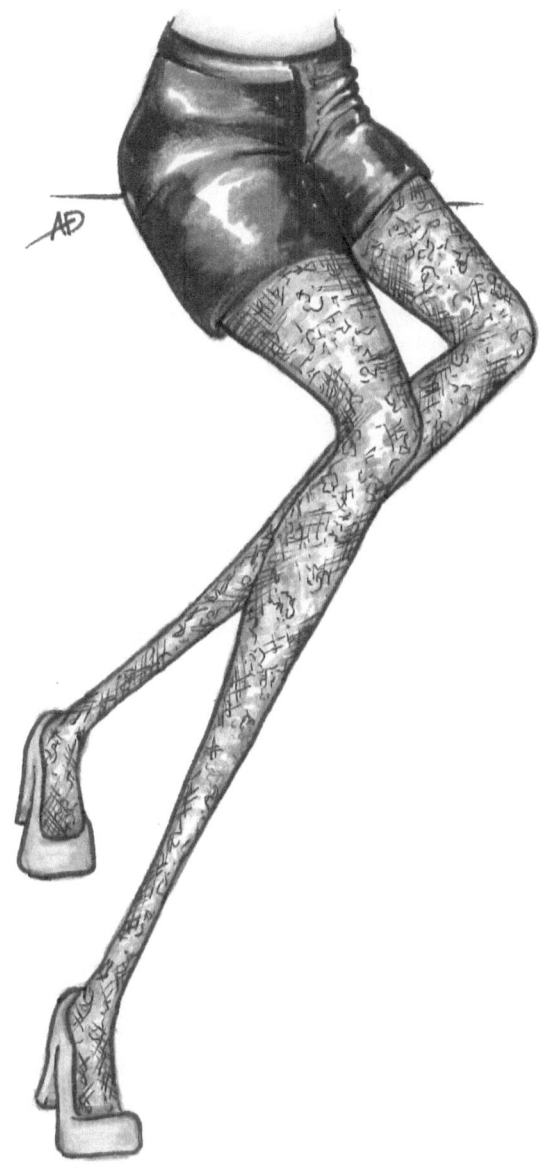

In contrast, if the lace only appears in the outfit minimally as a trim, set this demure detail off by accessorizing with shoes or handbags that have lace accents.

Layer It. Keep lace tunics and tops daytime savvy by layering them with a monochrome tank or slip. For example, a peek-a-boo black lace tee looks great over a black satin camisole. Don't forget that lace blouses are a fantastic way to set off a tailored suit, and ruffled lace tops take on a sophisticated air when worn with a pencil skirt and pumps.

Note: Invisible nude color underpinnings are best reserved for a more glamorous night look.

Body Balance. Lace immediately creates a focal point for the eye, so placement is essential. Lace tops and lace details along the neckline will bring the eye up and detract from full hips and tummy. Women looking to minimize a fuller upper body will benefit from chic lace skirts paired with a flattering heel.

Think Outside the Box. Add a modern twist by incorporating metallic lace into your outfit. Metallic lace dresses are perfectly paired with a simple heel or take on a cosmopolitan edge by pairing a metallic lace top with dark-wash denim. When wearing metallic lace and all-over lace styles, keep jewelry to a minimum.

Not so fashion forward? Lace details, accents, and trims are an easy way to seamlessly incorporate this look into a wardrobe. Lace adds textural dimension to any outfit and looks gorgeous when combined with a variety of fabrics. Think sleek leathers, sumptuous silks, and cozy tweeds.

Oh, and for those of you who raised a brow at the Elizabethan collar reference, this is not to be confused with the plastic collar worn by our furry four-legged friends after surgery. It is in fact a historical reference to the ruffs most popularly seen around the neck of Elizabeth I and other icons of the times. Not exactly water-cooler talk, but intriguing nonetheless. Who would have thought?

CHAPTER THIRTY-FOUR

Building Your Shoe Wardrobe

When building a gorgeous footwear wardrobe, style is equally as important as functionality. True, the color black goes with everything, but that doesn't mean that your comfy pair of black mukluks will. While it may not be practical for you to own fifty pair of shoes, you'll want to own the following essentials to allow for style versatility within your wardrobe. And *yes*, you can buy them all in black.

Flats: Even the most diehard heel loving fashionistas know that it's essential for every woman to have at least one pair of cute, comfortable flats. Think everyday slip-ons, pretty ballet flats, classic loafers and the like. Add a hint of your personal style through color and texture such as patent leather, metallic neutrals, fun prints and textured surfaces.

The Classic Pump: This is the universal answer to "what shoes should I wear?" for business meetings, dinners and formals. Their clean finish and low to mid heel height gives a fuss free approach to

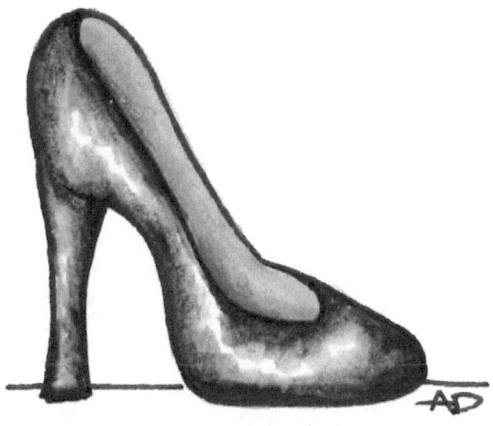

elegant style. At the very least, treat yourself to one quality pair in black. As you build your wardrobe, incorporate a neutral shade to set off your lighter colors.

The Sexy Heel: Whatever you call them, every woman should own a pair. Platforms, stilettos, peep toes, slinky or strappy –no matter your taste, *rock it*. This is the party shoe that celebrates your fun sexy side, so ensure the style encompasses your personality. Just be sure you can walk in them ;).

Trainers: Not to be confused with bulky gym shoes, trainers are sporty flats that can be worn every day. You will readily find them available in classic colors that will suit nearly every wardrobe. They have a comfy chic appeal when paired with jeans, tees, crops and sporty dresses.

Boots: A pair of boots in either black or brown

works well as a transitional footwear item. They can be worn with dresses, skirts, jeans, and leggings to name a fashionable few. The key to maximum wearability involves a little practicality. Select a heel height that you are comfortable in, along with a boot shaft height (how high the boot goes up the leg) that will seamlessly blend into the bulk of your wardrobe. You may find you will get more use out of a knee height boot with a low heel than an over the knee boot with a high stiletto heel. While both can be very stylish options, which will give you the most flexibility between work, play and weekend casual?

Important Footwear Heights

Heel Heights:

Flat: Under 1 inch

(*Under 2.5 centimeters*)

Low Heel: 1 inch to 1 ¾ inches

(*2.5 centimeters to 4.5 centimeters*)

Mid Heel: 2 inches to 2 ¾ inches

(*5 centimeters to 7 centimeters*)

High Heel: 3 inches and up

(*7.5 centimeters and up*)

Boot Shaft Heights:

Ankle Boots: 2 inches to 7 ¾ inches

(*5 centimeters to 19.5 centimeters*)

Mid-calf Boots: 8 inches to 13 ½ inches

(*20 centimeters to 34 centimeters*)

Knee-High Boots: 13 ¾ inches to 17 inches

(*35 centimeters to 43centimeters*)

Over the Knee Boots: 17 ¼ inches and up

(*44 centimeters and up*)

Quality and fit are priorities when shopping for shoe essentials. These styles are the building blocks of your footwear wardrobe and as a result they will receive the most wear. You owe it to yourself and the health of your feet to invest in a quality pair.

CHAPTER THIRTY-FIVE

Kitten Heels — The Perfect Sole-Mate

As much as I love shopping for new shoes, I definitely understand why it ends in frustration for so many women. It's usually a struggle between the practical footwear that looks suspiciously like a nursing shoe hybrid, or trendy styles that, judging by the four-inch heel, are completely non-functional.

However, your feet may be relieved to find that comfort and style have merged in the form of a delectably chic kitten heel.

And don't be fooled by the cute name. This mini-heel in the world of fashion-forward footwear is anything but short on style. From sexy sling-backs and peep-toes to tall boots and ankle booties, there are a variety of styles to choose from.

Girl Power. A kitten heel paired with a skirt is a fashionable way to wear this style of shoe. Think

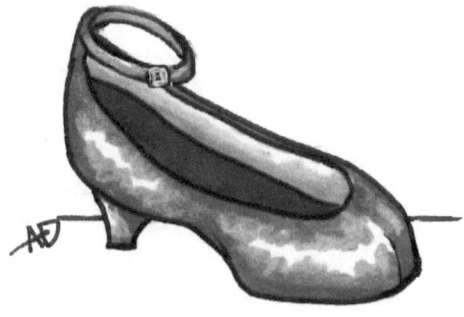

gorgeous A-lines, fluid circle skirts, and of course, the no-nonsense pencil skirt. Wear paired with a blouse or fitted knit for timeless, feminine style. Round toes are always a classic choice, while a pointy-toe kitten heel will work to visually slim the foot.

Texture. Although the cable-knit knee-high socks may be a stretch for the day to day, pay close attention to the concept. By pairing your kitten heel with a textured tight or trouser sock, you will add a splash of personality and style to your look. Even subtly ribbed hosiery in a complementary color will add a bit of intrigue to an otherwise mundane office look.

Lift. The subtle lift of the kitten heel looks fantastic with the cut of a full-leg trouser, creating the perfect balance between comfort and polish. The lower heel also makes this a practical choice to pair with boot-cut, straight-leg, and skinny denims for a comfy but cute day look. Do run your errands in style.

And speaking of running around…here are a few pointers on walking in heels.

Walking in heels is always a bit of a challenge, and for the newbie or those just tired of the teeter totter I recommend a kitten heel. The average height of a kitten heel is about one-and-a-half inches, providing a considerable step down from the average three-inch heels that line the sales floor. Simply stated? No need for intimidation. All that is required is a little practice.

Posture. Every story begins the same. Keep your back straight and your shoulders slightly back. This will promote an even distribution of your weight supported by the heel.

Three-Step Process. Take three steps forward. Why? Who ends in just one step? In order to become comfortable in new heels, however low, your body needs to adjust to the added height. Does it feel a little strange? This is normal. The muscles in your legs are being used in a way that is different from when you wear flats. As your body learns the memory of the heel, this feeling will dissipate.

Danger, Curves Ahead. When walking in heels, there is no reason to exaggerate the movement of your hips. Walk naturally, allowing your hips to move to the rhythm of your strides.

Dance Like Nobody's Watching. Yes, I am serious. Dancing around in heels is a fun way to adjust your body's movement in heels. Also the off-balance movement will train your body to quickly recover when on the verge of falling over. If you are in any way clumsy like I am, this is a necessity.

CHAPTER THIRTY-SIX

Stepping into Spring

Though we still wake to cool morning temps, the refashioning of the season is well underway. Comfy Uggs and fur-lined boots are being lovingly packed away and in their place will soon be easygoing flats, color-rich pumps, and cut-away ankle booties. Yes, spring has arrived.

Combine this with textured boat shoes, daring wedges, and lollipop-hued sandals and suddenly we have the makings for very happy feet.

Ballet Flats. Flirty and feminine style mavens will love the resurgence of floral details prevalent on the toes of sweet ballet flats. Organza rosettes, satin rosebuds, and colorful leather petals bring a refreshing transformation to casual separates. While these special touches create a delicate air, the materials used to create them shouldn't be.

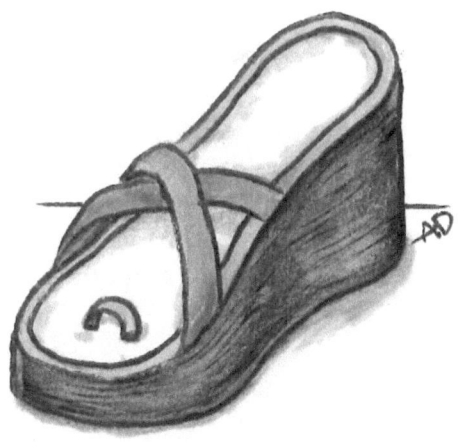

Floral trims and appliqués that are not reinforced with fusing or a backing will wear quickly over time, and you may find after only a few wears that your once-beautiful blossom has suddenly wilted. Check to ensure that textile embellishments are securely stitched down; otherwise, the pretty petals are only as good as the glue that holds them. Other lovely spring details to look for in store include bows, jewels, zippers, and neutral-tone lace.

Wedges. Wedges have returned to the fashion glossies in a parade of colors, textures, and styles. Seamlessly blending fashion and comfort, wedge styles are an ideal accompaniment to the sweeping dresses and skirts that epitomize the arrival of warmer weather. Wearers may find that one of the top benefits of wedges is that they are often easier to walk in than a high heel. The shape of the wedge provides additional support from the toe to the heel, assisting with balance. As with heels, wedges can be purchased in varying heights from high to low.

When accessorizing for wedge styles, keep scale in proportion. The shape of a wedge shoe is best balanced with looser-fitting apparel and fuller-leg jeans. If pairing a wedge with slim-cut apparel is a must, skip the chunky variety and opt for a slender wedge that will minimize the bulk.

Sandals. Metallic sandals give a luxe edge to the look of the warm weather, from casual shorts to sexy evening wear. A pair of gold, silver, or bronze sandals will gorgeously accent metallic evening dresses and sleek leather sandals take on an earthy air when worn with lightweight cotton dresses and colorful printed skirts.

Animal print always creeps its way into footwear in the form of reptile-printed gladiator sandals. These styles are ideal for dressing up casual trousers, denims, and crops. By pairing them with basic styles, these shoes add a fashionable pop that isn't too over the top. For an evening look, animal-printed gladiator sandals can be stylishly worn with solid-colored evening apparel in a flattering cut.

Other options to explore include perforated uppers, polished wooden heels, and neutral color combinations. Whatever your taste, be sure to accessorize your fancy-feet fashionably.

CHAPTER THIRTY-SEVEN

The Appeal of Eyewear

Sunglasses give a whole new meaning to the phrase "eye-catching style." Whether it's the cat-eye shades or the sleek aviator-style frames, they create a mood of glamour that hangs in the air. Choosing the best set of frames depends on the shape of your face as well as your personality. Here are a few tips on how to choose the right pair to enhance your look.

Aviators. The large lenses and unique frame of aviator sunglasses have made them a stylish favorite for venturing into the sunshine. Whether you're a diva, rebel or somewhere in the middle this chameleon frame will morph to suit both your day and evening looks. For a flattering appearance pay close attention to lenses size and frame color when purchasing.

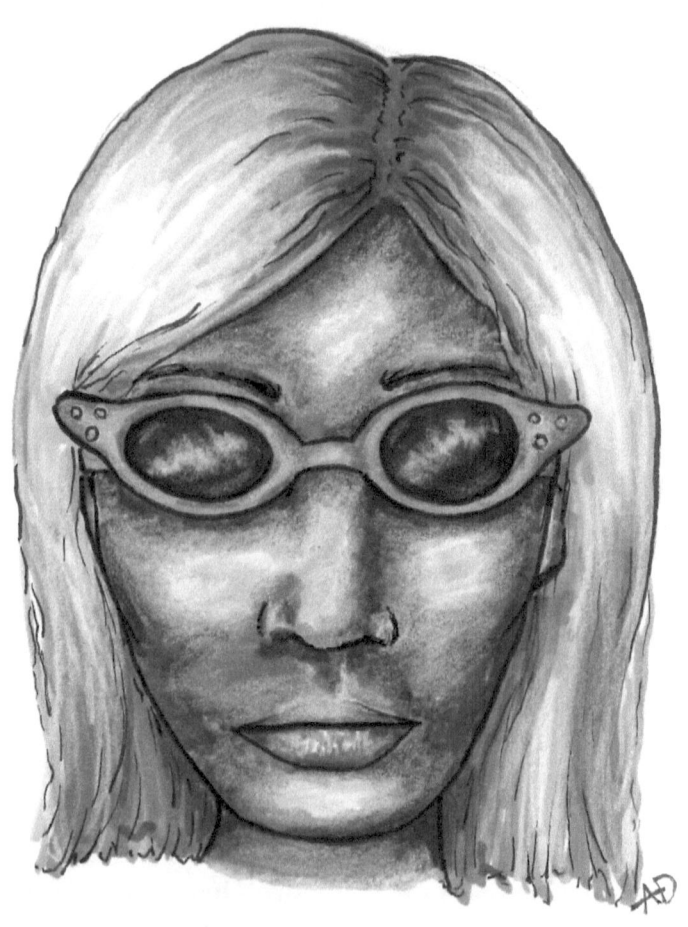

Cat Eye. Cat-eye sunglasses are a playful take on sexy eyewear. These fierce feline-inspired frames prance through sunny days, giving a retro twist to modern style. Characterized by the angled frames that tip up at both corners, these shades are novel for adding both style appeal and personality to an outfit. This season offers a playful selection of frames available in chic metallic, floral prints, and classic solids.

Circle. The clean, classic shape is as intriguing as the style icon that made these frames legendary. From tortoiseshell to thin, metal, rounded frames, the John Lennon–inspired sunglasses are a versatile addition that can be worn both casually with jeans and a tee or perfectly paired with a skirt or suit.

Oversize. On the larger end of the fashion accessory scale are oversized shades. Taking a style cue from the sixties and seventies, these big bold frames are notorious for infusing glamour into the eyewear scene. Avoid the bug-eye look by selecting the correct frame shape to suit your face. Try deviating from the norm and look for these signature A-list shades with a curved rectangular frame.

Wayfarer. This iconic fifties style touts a trapezoidal frame with structured arms for a fab finish. The longevity of the wayfarer style within the accessory arena proves that this frame is here to stay, so don't trouble yourself with trends. Available in a plethora of colors and prints the wayfarer frame can easily transition your outfit from casual to chic flawlessly.

A Note on Frames. Go from casual to chic in seconds with the perfect frames. When shopping for glasses for vision or the sun, you need the style that's most flattering on your face.

- o If you have an oval-shaped face, choose frames that are square or slightly rounded for your best look. This includes aviators, wayfarer and oversized frames.
- o If you have a round face, rectangular frames highlight your face the best. Other choices include the cat eye, wayfarer and oversized frames.
- o If you have a square face, circle frames are the best choice for the shape of your face. Additional style options include aviators and cat eye frames.
- o If you have a triangular face, look for frames with angled curves or an oval shape such as cat eye or wayfarer frames.

Sunglasses not only protect our eyes, they are also a fun way to make a statement about *who you are*.

CHAPTER THIRTY-EIGHT

Swimwear Help!

When the sunny days of summer finally arrive, the weather leaves many in a travel state of mind, including me. I mean, who wouldn't want to swap out hours in the office for lounging leisurely poolside or letting ocean waves soothingly wash your cares away? And while the decision to call in sick and fly south still remains an option, looking good in the stylish swimwear of summer is not. Luckily, swimwear designers continually serve up styles designed to effortlessly heat up the summer scene.

Dive into retro glamour with skirted and high-waist swimsuit styles that bring the pinup appeal of the past fashionably into the present. Pretty crochet-style swimwear offers a sweet escape from the norm. These intricate peek-a-boo styles exude creativity and textural intrigue for those looking to deviate from the same old same.

Fashion mavens who want to shimmer in the warm rays of the sun can create a dazzling display with pretty embellishments such as crystals, beading,

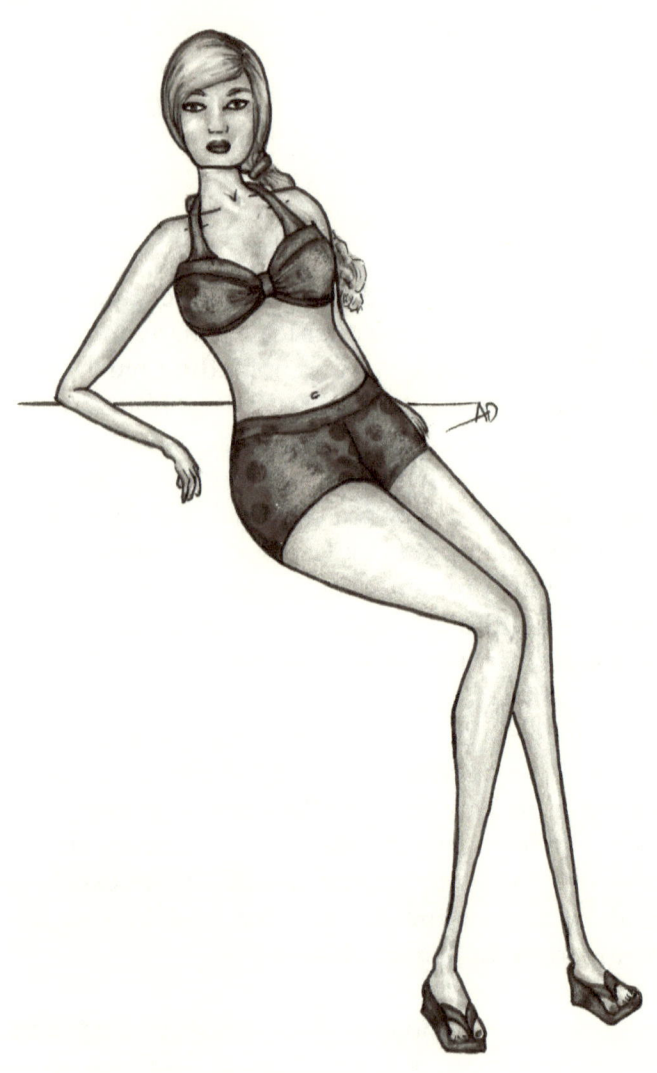

and studs. These divalicious details are spot on when it comes to dressing for the big resort and poolside parties of summer. Tribal prints compete for the spotlight with traditional tropical floral and wild things can always sink their teeth into a variety of animal prints from vivid peacock to exotic python.

These styles are available in several of silhouettes; choosing the right swimsuit will depend on the shape of your body. Below you will find quick tips to address the most popular swimwear shopping concerns.

Ruler. Bikinis and maillots with splashes of bold colors and prints play up slender silhouettes perfectly. Look for ruche details and built-in bras for added shape. If the full coverage of a one-piece swimsuit is more your style, shop for one that has details along the waist area. These details will give definition to your waistline and further enhance a slender silhouette. A belted bottom on a bikini or tankini will yield the same results.

Inverted Triangle. With this shape, wide shoulder straps are best as your upper body will benefit from the support in a bikini top or one-piece. Balance your shoulder line with your more narrow lower body by wearing a solid colored top with a playful printed bottom. Halter styles are a great choice and you can easily add visual appeal with side cut-out and asymmetric swimwear styles.

Pear. Curvy hips and bottoms look fabulous in playful swim dresses and two-piece styles that have a skirted bottom. The added length of the skirt minimizes the fullness of hips and thighs while providing additional coverage to your bottom. Make a point to avoid high-cut bottoms as this will exaggerate the width of fuller hips and thighs. Instead visually slim down with a sexy hipster bottom. Emphasize your upper body with cute bandeaus, halter styles and embellished tops.

Hourglass. Whether it's a polka dot bandeau, printed maillot or solid colored halter style this body shape can easily transition between most swimwear styles. Highlight the natural symmetry of your upper and lower body with coordinating two piece sets - avoid mismatching separates.

Apple. Flirty tankinis and gorgeous maillots are fashionable options for enhancing your silhouette. Swimwear styles with key hole cut outs at the bodice, v-necklines and single shoulder styles will bring the eyes up and visually detract from the fuller midsection of an apple. Empire styles and ruched panels along the midsection will have the same effect and high cut swimsuit bottoms are just the thing for showing off your more narrow lower body.

Tall and Petite. Taller women can break up a long torso with sexy cut-away swimwear styles and high-waist bikinis. In contrast, petite women can elongate a short torso with an empire band maillot and maximize leg lengths with high-cut bikini bottoms.

The Right Support. Fuller bustlines require an additional attention to detail when it comes to shoulder straps. Skip the skinny spaghetti straps and strings. Go instead for swimwear that has a wider shoulder strap to ensure the top of your swimsuit does not pull down and that your swim selection provides you with the support you need to sizzle in the sun. Swimwear with underwire cups will also assist with fit and support.

CHAPTER THIRTY-NINE

Outerwear Essentials

When you walk into a room, it's often your outerwear not the outfit beneath that gives viewers a first impression. For this reason it's important that your outerwear wardrobe provides you with workable style options for every occasion. Just as you wouldn't wear a hoodie to an elegant dinner over your dress, you don't want to be forced to wear your formal coat to a casual baseball game. To help get you started, below you will find a list of the most popular outwear essentials.

The Fitted Blazer. A fitted blazer is a wardrobe piece that can really save you in a style crunch. It automatically cleans up your work look for a sophisticated finish and is a no-brainer for job interviews. With its flattering cut a fitted blazer can be worn as part of a suit with trousers, jeans, skirts and over dresses. The key to looking good in this wardrobe essential is to purchase a style in the correct fit. Avoid boxy, shapeless styles as this will do nothing to flatter your figure. The shoulder seams should hit the edge of your shoulders and there should be ease in the lining for comfort when you bend your arms. If you only purchase one, opt for black, navy or grey.

The Trench Coat. The iconic trench coat serves as a great baseline for outerwear style. The silhouette defines your waist and eases over curves for fuss free fashion. It's a light weight coat suited for the coolness of spring and autumn. Trenches can be worn open and loose for a casual look or buttoned and belted for a smart finish. While the most common color for this coat is a neutral tan, don't be afraid to venture to red, yellow, hunter green, black or navy.

The Pea Coat. When the temperature dips to cold but it's not frosty enough for the goose down parka, your wool pea coat is an excellent option. It's a mid-weight coat that will provide added warmth without compromising style. Whether you prefer single or double breasted, military or swing style pea coats there are plenty of options to showcase your personality. The classic pea coat is universally flattering and is appropriate for all occasions, giving you a very fashionable advantage.

The Winter Coat. The snow and ice of winter typically call for a heavy weight coat that will insulate you from very cold temperatures. A quality body material and lining is essential with

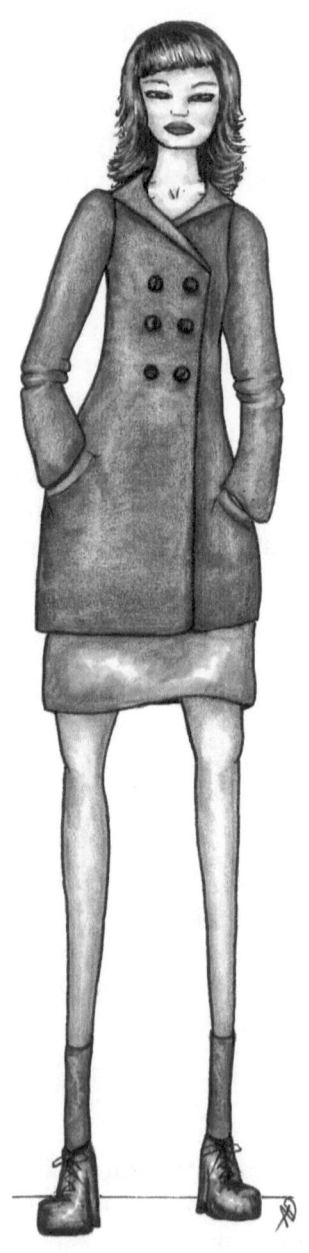

this type of coat, so shop wisely. Whether it's a puffer or a parka, there are countless designs available that incorporate both fashion and function. Belted and drawstring winter coats will give a feminine shape to your silhouette while quilting, ruching, chevron stitching and plush trims will keep you cute and cozy.

The Formal Coat. It's difficult to make a statement when your formal gown is topped off with a casual jacket. Special occasions require an elegant coat that will lay seamlessly over your dress or pantsuit for a stunning appearance For versatility opt for a ¾ to full length coat in black. The design should be clean, simple and cut to suit your shape.

Capes: The Essential Element for Invincible Style

There is something powerful about a beautiful, well-cut cape. Perhaps its leftover nostalgia from that pivotal childhood moment when my blanket became a cloak of super-girl invincibility or maybe a simple admiration of how a well-constructed cape can flatter just about any body type. Either way, this versatile cover-up has become the ultimate toss-on-and-go item for fall.

Thankfully, there are enough cape styles to suit every style personality, and better still it's a garment with maximum wear-ability that can be paired with both jeans and LBDs alike.

Voluminous Style. Wearing volume on both the upper and lower body can unfavorably add width to your silhouette. Keep your cape in proportion by wearing it with a fitted bottom such as a pencil skirt, slim cut trousers and denims, or leggings on your lower body.

If you decide to wear a fuller-leg pant or skirt, opt for a belted cape. The belt will bring the cape in at the waist, creating an hourglass silhouette that will ensure your shape is not lost in the folds of the fabric.

Short and Sweet. Shorter capes, known to the style masses as capelets, are a sweet way to top off cocktail dresses and holiday looks while fighting off the chill of cooler nights. In addition, the cropped cut of a capelet will visually elongate the torso for a leaner silhouette. Faux-fur capes are also popular in this cut and add an elegant finish to pretty LBDs. It's a cozy alternative to the shrug that looks great over strapless and sleeveless styles.

A Cut Above. When shopping for your stellar cape, you'll want to choose a style that suits your personality in a cut that flatters your body line. Cape styles with drape will visually add shape and curves to a straight silhouette. If you carry most of your weight along the upper body, avoid the tent effect with darts and seaming that will allow the fabric to fall over your curves in a flattering cut.

Note to petites: Avoid the longer cloak-style capes, as this will detract from your height.

Short on inspiration? Here are top cape looks for fall:

- o Utility-style capes look great with denims and tall, flat-heeled boots. Look for military

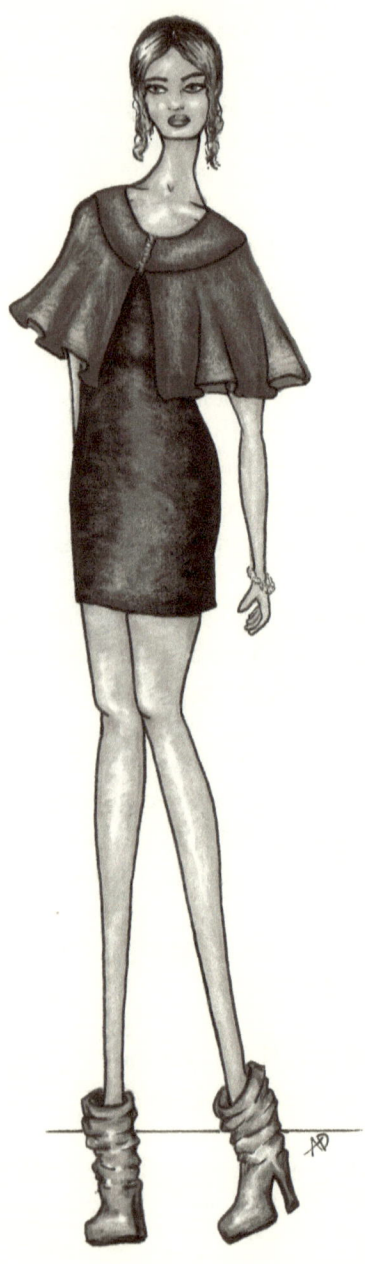

details such as metal buttons and epaulettes.

- o Structured wool capes over a fitted knit and fluid trousers lends to a commanding day look. Camel, gray, and navy are all versatile color options.
- o A fall cape worn over a blouse, skirt, opaque tights, and ankle booties paired with a structured cape or a draped shawl is a cute autumn look.

And while it won't give you superhuman strength or grant you invisibility when arriving late to work, this cozy cover-up will keep you wonderfully chic. *Superwomen unite.*

Outerwear: Perfecting the Puffer

A cold weather staple, padded (a.k.a. puffer) jackets and coats clearly can't be beat when it comes to staying warm and snug on cold winter mornings. I have also noted through the years that the padding of the down conveniently acts as a buffer between the human body and the pavement during icy tumbles on snowy days. But due to their added volume and construction, stylishly wearing puffer jackets can pose a problem for many fashion novices. However, with the correct cut, length, and fit, this cozy coat can quickly transform into a chic and trendy cold-weather look.

Give Shape to Your Puffer. Let's face it, with the added padding and typically boxy cuts, puffer jackets have a reputation for being anything but flattering. However, by belting your puffer jacket with a sleek belt, or purchasing a puffer that has the belt included, you will be well on your way to creating a svelte silhouette. The belt will work as a styling agent to bring the coat in at the waistline, creating waist definition as well as reducing the overall appearance of width. For maximum versatility and fit, opt for an elasticized belt.

The Tailored Puffer. If you are not so keen on belting up, a fitted puffer is a practical and cozy alternative. These jackets are cut to skim the body line and minimize bulk. This cut of puffer style look great in the cropped jacket styles, full-length puffers, as well as gilets.

Balance the Bulk. The key to looking slim and chic in your puffer jacket or coat is to balance the width of the puffer with your height. By wearing your puffer jacket with heels, whether it's a heeled winter boot or pump, you will lengthen the body line and bring balance to your silhouette.

Puffer Patterns. When selecting your perfect puffer jacket, pay close attention to the shape of the quilting. Square quilting is common and acceptable; however, if you prefer a more slimming effect, opt for a puffer jacket that has either diamond or herringbone-style quilting and paneling. The vertical V shape of these quilting styles will slim the body line for a flattering silhouette.

Lengthen the Line. Take a cue from après-ski chic and leave the collar of the puffer coat unzipped when temperatures allow. In doing

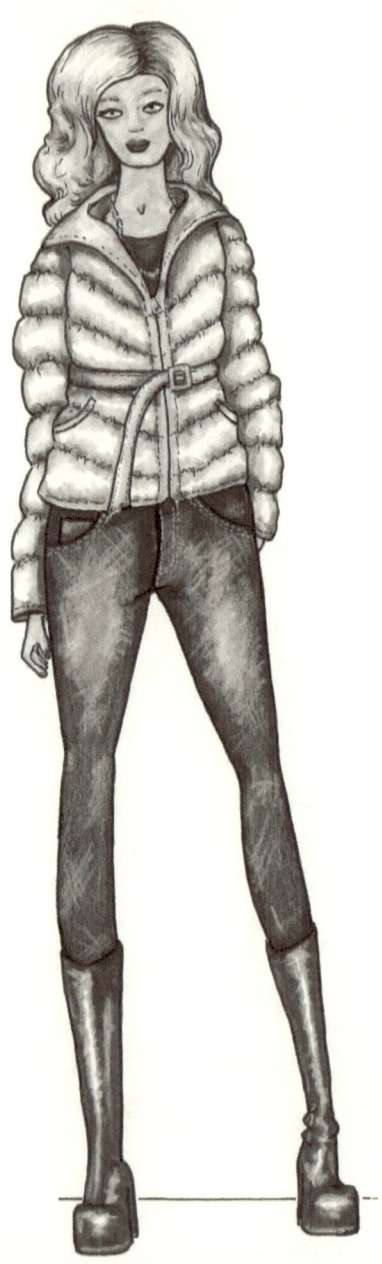

so, you will create a longer vertical line that will bring the eye up for a leaner affect.

Puffer Style. Creating a streamlined look with the puffer jacket boils down to selecting the right pairings. Choose lower-body garments with a lean fit. Think fitted boot-cut trousers, skinny jeans tucked into boots, and of course, the season's warm knit leggings. Fur- and shearling-trimmed puffer jackets are also great for added style and warmth during wear.

Note: Avoid baggy and voluminous lower-body garments, as this will result in the unflattering boxy silhouette that puffer styles are notorious for.

CHAPTER FORTY-TWO

Staying Warm in Style

Plush scarves, snuggly knits, and sleek winter gloves are key ingredients for staying fashionably warm in the colder months. And what better way to combat the gloom of Old Man Winter than by updating your wardrobe with colorful knits, playful Fair Isle patterns, and details made to dazzle even the coldest of nights during your holiday travels.

Scarves. Selecting the right scarf is a modern way to add style to your winter look while staying warm in the colder months ahead. This winter accessory is available in a variety of patterns, colors, and prints. With so many options available, selecting the right scarf is a matter of neck length and personality.

For those that have a shorter neck, avoid wrapping the scarf around your neck in multiple loops, as this will only add bulk and width to the neck area. Instead, loosely drape the scarf around the neck creating a U shape and let the ends hang down in front. Alternatively, tie the scarf in a loose knot that creates a V shape at the *base* of your neckline. This will expose enough of the neck for a balanced look.

If you have an average to long neck, simply wrap the scarf around your neck, letting the ends hang down or wear your scarf Parisian style with a folded loop. Start by folding the scarf in half, then wrap it around the neck from back to front and pull the ends through the loop that is created. Adjust the length and looseness of the scarf to your preference.

Gloves and Mittens. Evening gloves are a popular option for keeping both hands and arms warm during the holiday party season. Popular lengths range from just above the wrist to gloves worn fashionably just above the elbow. If you plan on wearing a strapless, short sleeve, or three-quarter-length sleeve, evening gloves are a solid option for updating a dress while adding texture and color to your holiday outfit.

However, when it comes to spending recreational time outdoors in the ice and snow, you will undoubtedly want a durable glove. If you have any intention of spending time in the snow, do your fingers a favor and opt for a waterproof glove. A standard glove will absorb the moisture from the snow and transfer it to your fingers, leaving your fingers and hands cold.

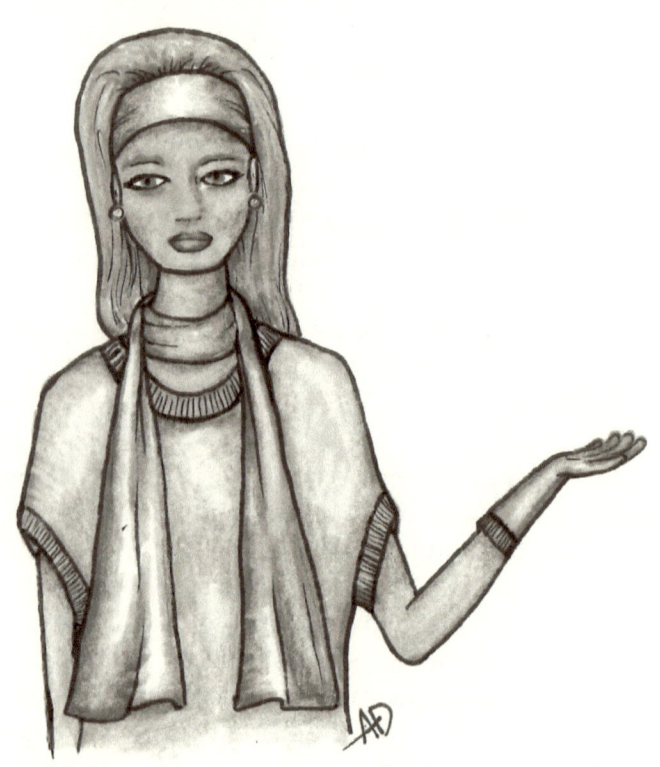

If you don't mind limited use of your fingers, mittens are often your best bet for keeping fingers warm during the cold season. Natural heat and insulation will be generated as a result of your four fingers being kept together in one snug place. Patterned and color-rich mittens are a sweet day look that work great with most casuals.

Knit Headbands. Hate hat hair? Knit headbands are a great way to keep both your head and ears warm without sacrificing style. Knit headbands can be easily incorporated into pretty hairstyles or worn in traditional outdoor style. When shopping for this item, you will find there are a variety of band widths, allowing flexibility when wearing over styled hair. For maximum wearability, pick up a few options in order to allow flexibility with your look.

To make a bold statement, look for chunky knit styles, which are perfect for accenting a sleek up-do. Designer style details such as bows, floral shapes, and fur will also add a special accent to your look. If a casual look is more your style, select a headband that has a thinner, fine-gauge knit designed to lay flat against your hair.

Whether you venture to the great beyond to visit relatives or stay local to enjoy seasonal cheer, use these top winter accessories to keep your wardrobe cozy and chic.

Five Tips to Help You Avoid Looking Frumpy

Just as you don't have to be a style icon to look stylish, you don't have to spend a fortune on the trendiest clothes in order to avoid looking frumpty-dumpty. Here are some basic style tips that can help:

1. **Wear clothes that fit.** This may seem obvious, but ill-fitting clothes are the biggest contributor to a frumpy look. For most women, large, baggy, or unstructured styles will result in a frumpy look, so look for structure and seaming to enhance your feminine silhouette.

2. **The perfect skirt length.** Every woman has an ideal skirt length—the perfect length that looks great on her every time. Typically, this length is either just above or just below the knee. Consult your friends and the mirror to determine yours, and have most of your skirts adjusted to this length (exceptions would be miniskirts or longer evening gowns).

3. **Keep your hairstyle current.** Update your hairstyle at least every five years. The change doesn't have to be dramatic — sometimes a slight change in length, layering, or color can make such a big difference.

4. **Consider your shoes.** Don't wear old shoes until they fall apart. Worn-out shoes can look really frumpy, as can shoes that are out of style. So keep it fresh!

5. **Accessories matter.** Make sure your everyday accessories such as glasses and watches are in style. Earrings, necklaces, purse, and scarf styles can change quickly, so while they are not a necessity, they do offer a great way for updating a look when needed for a pop of modernity.

All of this being said, keep in mind that what may look frumpy on one person may look really great on another. Try different options, and if you're not sure, ask for opinions.

Following these simple steps can go a long way in helping you stay up to date and looking fabulous.

How to Transition Summer Clothing into Your Fall Wardrobe

Whether you're a stay-at-home mom or a woman on the go, the start of fall often means changing out those summer clothes for some that are more appropriate for cooler weather. While this can be a fun excuse for a shopping spree, there are many summer pieces that can actually be transitioned to your fall wardrobe. Repurposing some of your summer clothes in this manner can help lower your new fall wardrobe costs.

When looking through your summer clothes to see what you can keep out for a few more months, pull out all the basics. This includes everything from tank tops to simple dresses. Just because the weather is too cold to wear a tank top in late October does not mean that you can't make it fall chic under a blazer. Even casual summer tops can be turned into business casual for the office by layering it with a nice jacket. Belt your favorite summer dress and add a darker cardigan or blazer with a pair of leggings or knee socks. In fact, if you have been wearing leggings during the summer, be sure to keep out the neutral colors for fall. Finish off the leggings or dress with boots for a funky fall chic look.

In terms of colors and designs, fall hues are generally warm earth tones such as browns, greens, and oranges. When selecting the summer clothes that you're going to keep out, stick with pieces that have rich colors to match the standard fall tones, such as a burgundy or navy top.

Don't worry about your summer clothing being too thin to wear in the fall because you can layer with a thicker fall piece. Adding a vest, blazer, or scarf to a summer blouse not only makes it fall-ready but ensures that you are warm enough to wear it to a bonfire or other fall event.

CHAPTER FORTY-FIVE

Stellar Style: How to Organize Your Clothing and Accessories

Shirts dangling from hangers, shoes strewn across the floor, and jackets bunched together in a closet are perfect if your style is desperately sifting through clothes in the morning and tossing on whatever you can find after giving it a good shake. But if it's peace and solace you're after, here are a few basic tips to assist you in creating a wardrobe that will save you time and energy and keep you looking your best.

Did you ever notice how much time is saved while shopping when you select a blouse you love and right next to it is a coordinating pencil skirt? Grouping outfits together in the closet will eliminate the hassle of searching for the right garment to pair with another, particularly on mornings when time is scarce. And if you suffer from that thing that pulls you out of bed every morning commonly referred to as a job, you will appreciate any extra time that you can save. Toss in a few kids and a pet and you'll *really* appreciate this.

Grouping. If you have a shirt that looks great with a certain pair of trousers and blazer, group them together. Once the first outfit is complete, put together another outfit and so on. Any leftover items should be grouped by garment type (e.g., pants, skirts) then by color for easy reference.

Shoes should be stored on a shoe rack or hanger or in shoes boxes that are either clear or have a photo on the front of the box for easy identification.

Sweaters can be folded and organized on shelves by color.

Generally, outerwear is the most bulky of items stored in the closet. These garments should be grouped together by length then color at the end of the rail.

Accessories. All belts should be hung together for quick reference. This can be done by purchasing hooks, using nails, or securing them on a strong hanger.

Loose items such as wraps and scarves should be placed on hangers, secured by a clamp, clothes pins, or draped from a hook.

Hats are best stored in boxes and placed on shelves.

All out-of-season items can easily be stored in clear plastic under-the-bed storage bins. This will help to eliminate excess clutter in the closet.

Final Touches. Place a sachet in your closet for a light fragrance that's fresh and inviting.

Following the above steps will assist you in creating a wardrobe that's organized and time efficient. It will also help you to visually distinguish between what you need for future purchases and what you don't.

Tying It All Together

As you read this final chapter, you should have an understanding of how your beauty stems from within, the importance of supporting yourself through life's challenges and the knowledge of fashion fundamentals to build your wardrobe.

If who you are is the building block of your beauty, it's only natural that you pause and review all that you have learned about yourself through completing the Beauty Brainstorms. In what ways did you surprise yourself? What important lessons have you learned?

As with any new relationship, be patient with yourself as you continue to develop your inner beauty. Remember that with each obstacle comes an opportunity to seek out the lesson and become a stronger woman.

Approach your wardrobe with the understanding that even though your closet may not be filled with the latest couture, every garment you wear is priceless. Why? Because every pattern, cut and color signifies *who you are*.

These are the seeds of your beauty and with each day, may they lovingly grow.

~Lakeysha-Marie

Twitter: @seedsofbeauty

About the Author

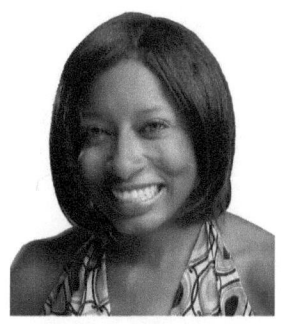

Author Lakeysha-Marie Green is no stranger to tackling style dilemmas. A fashion stylist and former women's fit technologist, her extensive experience in the fashion industry taught her the importance of fit, fashion, and effortless style. Her penchant for creativity led to her work in editorial magazines, international film premieres, and advertising.

Lakeysha-Marie holds a degree in Fashion Design & Merchandising, with continued coursework in styling & photography from the London College of Fashion.

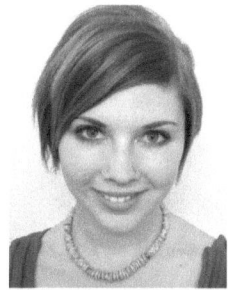

Illustrator Alyse DeCavallas is a Southern California based artist and technical fashion designer. She has studied fine arts at CalArts and Parson's School of Design, as well as received a degree in Fashion Design from FIDM in Los Angeles. She has worked in the fashion industry since 2007, as a patternmaker, manufacturer, and technical designer.

Acknowledgements

I would like to thank the following family members, friends and colleagues for their suggestions and valuable feedback : my parents Dale and Dee, my sister Tawana, my brothers Dale and Brent. Erin Meyer, Crystal L. Gardner, Lloyd Barrett, Erroll Perkins, Jennifer Ruby, Heather Golden, Marisa Ligons and Alyse DeCavallas.

…And a special thank you to You, the reader.

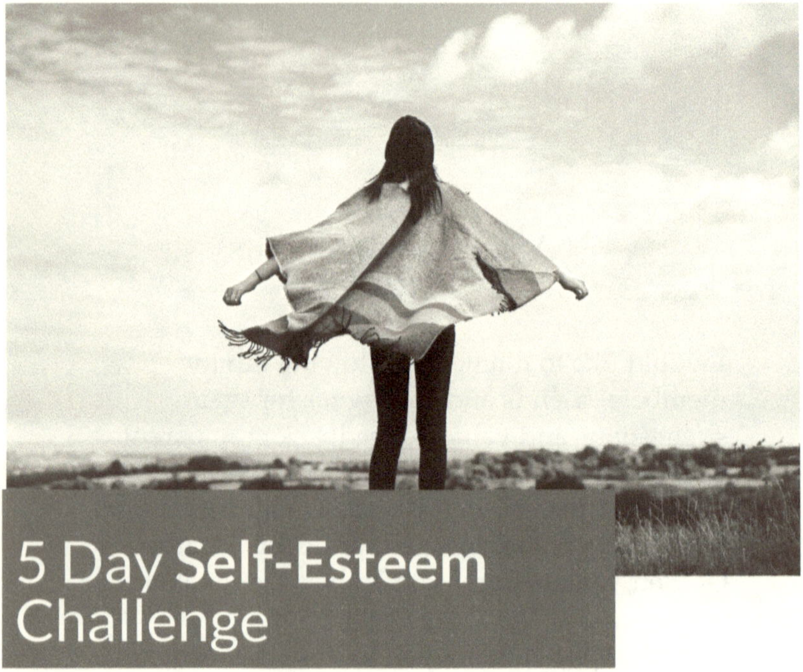

5 Day **Self-Esteem** Challenge

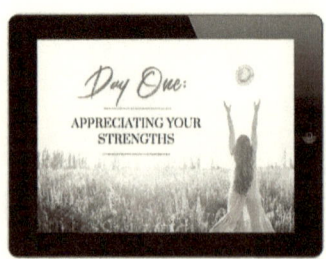

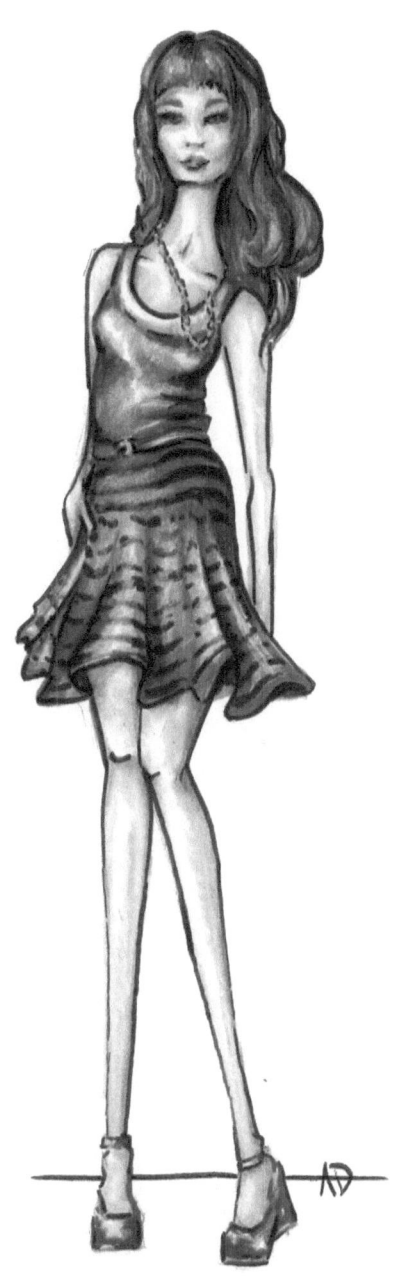